THE
CORONAVIRUS
PREVENTION
HANDBOOK

101 SCIENCE-BASED TIPS THAT COULD SAVE YOUR LIFE

Chief Editor **Wang Zhou, MD,**

Chief Physician of Wuhan Center for Disease Control and Prevention

Foreword by Nanshan Zhong, Translated by Shan Zhu, Qing Chen, Jun Li

T0058065

SKYHORSE PUBLISHING

Chief Editor: Wang Zhou
Reviewed by Yongjian Xu
Foreword by Nanshan Zhong
Translated by Shan Zhu, Qing Chen, Jun Li

Visit our website at www.skyhorsepublishing.com.

10 9 8 7 6 5 4 3

Library of Congress Cataloging-in-Publication Data is available on file.

Cover design by Brian Peterson
Cover images: Getty Images

Print ISBN: 978-1-5107-6241-1
Ebook ISBN: 978-1-5107-6244-2

Printed in the United States of America

Words from the Translators

In this era of globalization, non-stop movements of humans and goods make no country immune to the potential threat of epidemics. Since 2003, emergent contagious diseases such as the avian influenza, Middle East respiratory syndrome, SARS, and Ebola reminded us human beings once and again of the grave threat that they pose to the human health and the economic and social security.

While the spread of COVID-19 is gradually being contained in China, the world is facing several new hot spots such as Japan, South Korea, Iran, and Italy. So, dissemination of the knowledge and know-hows of the prevention and control of the epidemic is urgent and essential not only for China but also for the world.

In the early days of the outbreak, China promptly shared its understanding of the virus with the world through the World Health Organization. Tested and tempered by the viral epidemic such as SARS epidemic, the frontline professionals and experts at the "epicenter"—Wuhan, decided to share their invaluable experiences and lessons drawn from the current outbreak as well as during their careers in China and various countries in the form of the Handbook of Prevention and Control of COVID-19 in Chinese.

To prepare non-Chinese speakers for personal protection, contain the global spread of 2019-nCoV, and share Chinese solutions to the epidemic with the world, the publishing house invited the Translators Association of China to promote the translation program. Under their guidance, the Center for Medical Language Service of Guangdong University of Foreign Languages was nominated for this mission and, shortly recruited the volunteers who worked with an all-out effort and completed the work in time.

This book, especially the measures that individuals and communities can adopt at the time of an outbreak, might serve as an important source of information on the prevention and control of both the present and future epidemics. Even if China's experiences do not apply to all countries in the same manner, they should serve as valuable references.

The intended readership of this book includes health professionals and the public, and archiving of the book may be suggested for public and professional, academic libraries. Readers can find topics of their interest in the contents page and jump directly to the relevant pages without finishing the preceding ones.

Despite our best efforts to review and proofread, unintended errors may remain in the book. The responsibility lies with all of us, and comments and suggestions for the improvement of translation are much appreciated.

Translation Team
February 2020

Those who contribute to the English version are as follows.

Translation Counselors
Dr. Ping Yang, Translators Association of China
Ruilin Li, School of Interpreting and Translation Studies, Guangdong University of Foreign Studies

Translators
Shan Zhu, School of Foreign Studies, China University of Petroleum(Huadong)

Dr. Qing Chen,Center for Medical Language Service, Guangdong University of Foreign Studies

Dr. Jun Li, School of Medical Humanities, Peking University

Gao Chen, Guangzhou Bon-lion Tech Co., Ltd.

Kuan-Hung Chen, First-Affiliated Hospital, Sun Yat-Sen University

Shane Lau, Chinese University of Hong Kong

Fengyuan Yang,State Key Laboratory of Respiratory Disease, Guangzhou Medical University

Li Li, Nanjing University of Chinese Medicine

Lin Shen, Guangdong university of Foreign Studies

Bilingual Proofreader
Dr. Jongdae Lee, State Key Laboratory of Respiratory Disease, Guangzhou Medical University

Contents

Editorial Board

Introduction to Editors-in-Chief

Wang Zhou, MD, Chief Physician (Level 2) of Wuhan Center for Disease Control and Prevention. Senior Visiting Scholar, University of Pennsylvania, 2005 to 2006.

Funded by the "213 Talent Project" by Wuhan Municipal People's Government in 2003;

Funded by "Huanghe Talent Program" by Wuhan Municipal Committee of the Communist Party of China in 2015;

Professor, Huazhong University of Science and Technology and Wuhan University

Director, Chinese Association for STD and AIDS Prevention and Control;

Executive director, Hubei Preventive Medicine Association,

Vice chairman and secretary-general, Wuhan Branch, Chinese Preventive Medicine Association;

Director, Wuhan Association for STD/AIDS Prevention and Treatment;

Member of editorial board, Chinese Journal of Preventive Medicine and Chinese Journal of Viral Diseases.

Rich experience in epidemiology and control of contagious diseases;

Principal investigator, research projects funded by the National Institutes of Health (US), the Bill & Melinda Gates Foundation, the National Health Commission of China, and the Hubei Health Commission

Winner of four Science and Technology Progress Awards of Hubei Province or Wuhan City;

First/corresponding author of more than 50 academic journal articles (over 20 in SCI/SSCI journals).

Qiang Wang, MD, professor of the School of Medicine of the Wuhan University of Science and Technology;

Visiting scholar of MD Anderson Cancer Center, the University of Texas (2015-2016);

Standing committee member and secretary-general, Committee of Cancer and Microecology, China Anti-Cancer Association;

Deputy chairman, Blood Section, Rehabilitation Branch, Chinese Anti-Cancer Association;

Standing committee member, Immunology Branch, China Association of Chinese Medicine;

Deputy director, Youth Committee, China Association of Chinese Medicine;

Standing committee member, Tenth Council, Hubei Society for Immunology;

Member, Sixth Committee, Microbiology and Immunology Branch, Hubei Medical Association.

Rich experience in the immunology of infectious diseases, tumor microenvironment, and preventive interventions on AIDS among college students in China;

Principal investigator of research projects funded by the Ministry of Education of China, and the Departments of Science and Technology, and of Education of Hubei province;

Winner of a Science and Technology Progress Award of Hubei province;

First/corresponding author of more than 20 academic journal articles (10 in SCI/SSCI journals); editor-in-chief of three textbooks.

Ke Hu Professor and Director of the Second Department of Respiratory and Critical Care Medicine of Renmin Hospital of Wuhan University (Hubei Renmin Hospital), chief physician, and doctoral supervisor.

Principal investigator of four projects funded by the National Natural Science Foundation of China and one sub-project of the National Key Research and Development Project "Research on di-

agnosis and treatment of COPD complications and comorbidities".
First or corresponding author of over 100 academic journal papers.

Has participated in the clinical treatment of many public health emergencies in Hubei Province since the SARS outbreak in 2003.

Zaiqi Zhang, doctor of internal medicine, postdoctor of emergency medicine, MBA, chief physician, professor, doctoral supervisor, and member of the CPC Committee and vice president of Hunan University of Medicine.

Deputy director, Committee of Health Emergency, Chinese Research Hospital Association

Deputy director, Committee of Emergency Resuscitation, Chinese Medical Doctor Association

Deputy director and deputy manager, Committee of Disaster Medicine and Committee of Chemical Injury Treatment, Chinese Association of Integrative Medicine

Vice director and vice chairman, Committee of Modernization of Medicine and Clinical Translation, China National Medical Association, and director, Committee of Disaster Medicine, Hunan Association of Chinese and Integrative Medicine.

Principal investigator of over 32 national and local research projects,

Author of 82 academic journal articles in Chinese and English;

Winner of 12 provincial and local research awards;

Editor-in-chief of *Diagnosis and Treatment in Clinical Emergency, Clinical Treatment of Critical Conditions, Disaster and First Aid, Formulary of Practical Therapy*, among others.

Foreword

The novel coronavirus pneumonia (COVID-19) that was first reported from Wuhan, China has spread all around China and even to other countries in the world. Confirmed cases of COVID-19 have mounted to a number far exceeding that of SARS in 2003, and its mortality is not negligible. Realizing its "human-to-human" transmission capability, the World Health Organization identified it as a Public Health Emergency of International Concern on January 31, 2020. These facts are enough to illustrate the severity and complexity of the outbreak.

Given the fact that no effective medicine is available for viral infectious diseases, the preventive measures including control of the source of infection, early detection of patients, cutting off transmission, and protecting susceptible population are paramount. Although medical institutions and workers are the main force fighting the disease, public participation is also indispensable for a rapid epidemic control. Therefore, it is extremely important to disseminate the relevant information to the public.

With that in mind, Professor Wang Zhou of the Wuhan Center for Disease Control and Prevention organized a panel of experts to compile this Handbook about the overview of the coronaviruses and its transmission, detection and treatment of the disease, precautions for individuals and public places, and basics about contagious diseases. With graphic illustrations and plain language, this book is intended to serve as a systematic introduction to the scientific knowledge on COVID-19.

The speed and scope of spread of COVID-19 makes the publication of this book urgent. I believe it will play an essential role in popularizing relevant knowledge, raising awareness of disease prevention and control, and preventing social panic. I am more than delighted to write the preface.

Nanshan Zhong
January 2020

Preface

In December 2019, scores of pneumonia cases with unknown causes presenting with fever, fatigue, coughing, and breathing difficulties as the main symptoms occurred in Wuhan within a short period of time. The Chinese governments and health departments at all levels placed great importance on the disease and immediately enacted measures for disease control and medical care, and directed research institutions to initiate investigations, treatments and collaborative research. The pathogen of the disease was quickly identified as a novel coronavirus, which was subsequently confirmed by the World Health Organization (WHO). The WHO named the virus 2019-nCoV while the International Committee on Taxonomy of Viruses (ICTV) coined it SARS-Cov-2; and the pneumonia caused by the viral infection was called novel coronavirus pneumonia (COVID-19) by WHO.

This handbook aims to improve the understanding of the disease among the public as well as people in relevant professions, and to provide a guidance on personal preventive measured to reduce the transmission risks. For these purposes, the Wuhan Center for Disease Control & Prevention promptly organized specialists in contagious disease control, researchers in pathogenic organisms and immunology, and front-line clinical experts at tertiary hospitals to compile THE CORONAVIRUS PREVENTION HANDBOOK. The book consists of six parts: 1) overview of the coronaviruses, 2) transmission of coronaviruses, 3) COVID-19 detection, diagnosis and treatment, 4) personal precautions, 5) precautions in public places, and 6) basics on contagious diseases. It addresses the concerns of the public on COVID-19. If we are united in the face of adversities and execute epidemic prevention measures based on scientific evidence, we will undoubtedly win this battle.

In the compilation of the handbook, we referred to relevant published literature and official reports. The editorial board sincerely apologizes for the absence of citation trails or references due to the time constraint. If there are any problems or errors with the content, please feel free to contact us. Your comments and suggestions would be much appreciated.

Editorial Board
January 2020

I. Overview of Coronaviruses

1. What are viruses associated with respiratory infections?

"Viruses associated with respiratory infections" refer to the viruses that invade and proliferate in the epithelial cells of the respiratory tracts that could cause respiratory and systemic symptoms.

2. What are the common viruses associated with respiratory infections?

Viruses from the family Orthomyxoviridae (influenza viruses), the family Paramyxoviridae (paramyxoviruses, respiratory syncytial virus, measles virus, mumps virus, Hendra virus, Nipah virus and human metapneumovirus), the family Togaviridae (Rubella virus), the family Picornaviridae (rhinovirus), and the family Coronaviridae (SARS coronavirus) are the common respiratory viruses. In addition, adenovirus, reovirus, coxsackie virus, ECHO virus, herpes virus, etc. can also cause infectious respiratory diseases.

3. What are coronaviruses?

Coronavirus are unsegmented single-stranded positive-strand RNA viruses. They belong to the order Nidovirales, the family Coronaviridae, and the subfamily Orthocoronavirinae, which is divided into α, β, γ, and δ genera according to their serotypic and genomic characteristics. Coronaviruses belong to the genus Coronavirus of the family Coronaviridae. It is named after the wreath-shaped protrusions on the envelope of the virus.

4. What are the shape and structure of coronaviruses?

Coronaviruses have an envelope encasing the RNA genome), and the virions (the whole viruses) are round or oval, often polymorphic, with a diameter of 50 to 200 nm. The novel coronavirus is 60 to 140 nm in diameter. The spike protein is located on the surface of the virus and forms a rod-like structure. As one of the main antigenic proteins of the virus, the spike protein is the main structure used for typing. The nucleocapsid protein encapsulates the viral genome and can be used as a diagnostic antigen.

5. How are coronaviruses classified?

Most coronaviruses infect animals. Currently, three types of coronaviruses have been isolated from humans: Human Coronaviruses 229E, OC43, and SARS coronavirus (SARS-CoV). There are 6 types of coronaviruses previously known to infect humans. 229E and NL63 (of alphacoronaviruses), OC43 (of betacoronaviruses), HKU1, Middle East Respiratory Syndrome Coronavirus (MERS-CoV), and Severe Acute Respiratory Syndrome Coronavirus (SARS-CoV).

Recently, a novel coronavirus was isolated from the lower respiratory tract of patients in Wuhan, who were suffering from pneumonia due to unknown causes (The World Health Organization (WHO) called it 2019-nCoV while the International Committee on the Taxonomy of Viruses (ICTV) named it SARS-CoV-2. It was subsequently confirmed that the virus is capable of human-to-human transmission.

This novel coronavirus is very similar in terms of the genome sequences to six previously discovered coronaviruses. An analysis of their genetic sequence homology revealed that the new virus has many similarities with SARS-CoV. This novel coronavirus is now classified as a beta-coronavirus.

6. Which wild animals carry coronaviruses?

Many wild animals carry pathogens and are potential transmission vectors of certain contagious diseases. Bats, civets, badgers, bamboo rats, and wild camels, etc. are known hosts of coronaviruses.

The outbreak of novel coronavirus pneumonia originated in Wuhan has many similarities to the SARS outbreak in Guangdong back in 2003: both began in the winter; the initial cases were traced to contacts with fresh, live animals in a market; both were caused by a previously unknown coronavirus.

Due to the similarity of the genomic sequences between the novel coronavirus and a coronavirus found in bats, which is 85% or higher, it is speculated that bats are the natural hosts of the novel coronavirus. Like the SARS coronavirus that caused the outbreak in 2003, the novel coronavirus is likely to have intermediate hosts between bats and humans yet unknown to us.

Therefore, one should refrain from consumption of uninspected wild animals or uncooked food such as meat sold by roadside sellers.

7. How do coronaviruses transmit from animals to humans?

Many coronaviruses that infect humans could be found in bats, which are natural reservoirs of coronaviruses. Bats are likely to be the original host of the novel coronavirus. Transmission from bats to humans might have occurred after mutation via an intermediate host(s). The genomic sequence analysis showed a more than 85% homology between the novel coronavirus and a coronavirus in bats. However, there are several other possible intermediate hosts between bats and humans, which have not been confirmed yet. Animal-to-human or human-to-human transmission relies mainly on two routes: contacts and droplets.

The coronaviruses that are currently known to cause pneumonia in humans include HKU1, SARS-CoV, MERS-CoV, and 2019-nCoV.

8. How resilient are coronaviruses in different environments?

Viruses generally can survive for several hours on smooth surfaces. If the temperature and humidity permit, they can survive for several days. The novel coronavirus is sensitive to ultraviolet rays and heat. Sustained heat at 132.8°F for 30 minutes, ether, 75% alcohol, chlorine-containing disinfectants, peracetic acid, chloroform, and other lipid solvents can effectively inactivate the virus. Chlorhexidine (also known as chlorhexidine gluconate) also effectively inactivates the virus.

The survival time of the novel coronavirus 2019-nCoV at different environmental temperatures is as follows.

Different environments	Temperature	Survival time
Air	50 ~ 59°F	4 hours
	77°F	2 ~ 3 minutes
Droplets	<77°F	24 hours
Nasal mucus	132.8°F	30 minutes
Liquid	167°F	15 minutes
Hands	68 ~ 86°F	<5 minutes
Non-woven fabric	50 ~ 59°F	<8 hours
Wood	50 ~ 59°F	48 hours
Stainless steel	50 ~ 59°F	24 hours
75% alcohol	Any temperature	<5 minutes
Bleach	Any temperature	<5 minutes

9. How virulent is the 2019-nCoV?

Common coronaviruses mainly infect adults or older children, causing the common cold. Some strains can cause diarrhea in adults. These viruses are mainly transmitted by droplets, and can also be spread via the fecal-oral route. The incidence of corona virus infection is prevalent in winter and spring. The incubation period for coronaviruses is usually 3 to 7 days.

2019-nCoV is a coronavirus that underwent antigenic mutations. The incubation period of the virus is as short as 1 day but generally considered to be no longer than 14 days. But it should be noted that some reported cases had an incubation period of up to 24 days.

To measure the degree of harm caused by a virus, both infectivity and lethality should be considered. The new coronavirus is highly-infectious and can be fatal, but its lethality has not been determined at present.

10. Can humans develop immunity to 2019-nCoV?

Scientific data on the level and the duration of protective immune antibodies produced in patients after infection of the novel coronavirus remain scarce. In general, the protective antibodies (immunoglobulin G, IgG) against a virus can be produced two weeks or so after an infection, and may exist for several weeks to many years, preventing re-infection of the same virus after recovery. Currently efforts are underway to test whether recently recovered from 2019-nCoV infection carry protective antibodies in the blood.

11. What is Severe Acute Respiratory Syndrome (SARS)?

Severe acute respiratory syndrome (SARS) is a disease caused by SARS-CoV. The main symptoms of SARS include fever, cough, headache, muscle pain, and other symptoms of respiratory infection. Most SARS patients recover with or without medical treatment. Its fatality rate is about 10%; those over 40 years of age or with underlying diseases (such as coronary heart disease, diabetes, asthma, and chronic lung diseases) are most at risk to develop the fatal disease.

12. What is Middle East Respiratory Syndrome (MERS)?

Middle East Respiratory Syndrome is caused by MERS-CoV. It was first reported in middle-eastern countries including Saudi Arabia, United Arab Emirates etc. People who are infected by MERS-CoV can develop acute respiratory distress syndrome (ARDS), while the most common manifestations being fever with tremors, coughing, shortness of breath, sore muscles and gastrointestinal symptoms such as diarrhea, nausea, vomiting or stomachache. Severe cases are featured by respiratory failure which require mechanical ventilation and supportive treatment in ICU. Some patients developed organ failures, especially renal failure and sceptic shock which eventually led to death. The case fatality rate is about 40%. Since the onset of the first MERS case in September 2012 until May 2015, MERS cases have been reported in 25 countries around the world, posing a serious threat to public health.

13. What is novel coronavirus? Why has it become epidemic?

The newly discovered coronavirus is a mutated novel coronavirus (β genus), which is named 2019-nCoV by the WHO and SARS-CoV-2 by the ICTV. On January 10, 2020, genomic sequencing of the first sample of 2019-nCoV was completed, and the viral genomic sequences of five more samples were subsequently announced.

Due to the antigenic mutations that made this corona virus new to humans, the general population lacks immunity against the new strain. Furthermore, there are more than one routes of transmission for this virus. These factors resulted in the novel coronavirus becoming epidemic.

II. Transmission of 2019-nCoV

14. What is community-acquired pneumonia?

Community-acquired pneumonia (CAP) refers to infectious pulmonary parenchymal pneumonia (including in the alveolar wall, which belongs to the lung interstitium in a broad sense) contracted outside the hospital setting, including pneumonia from known pathogens presenting after admission within its average incubation period.

15. What are the diagnostic criteria for community-acquired pneumonia?

The diagnostic criteria for community-acquired pneumonia are:
(1) Onset in community.
(2) The clinical manifestations of pneumonia are as follows.
- New presentation of cough, sputum, or exacerbation of existing respiratory diseases, with or without purulent sputum/chest pain/ dyspnea/hemoptysis.
- Fever.
- Pulmonary consolidation and/or presence of wet rales.
- WBC (white blood cells) counts higher than 10×10^9/L or lower than 4×10^9/L, with or without a left shift of neutrophil nucleus (a sign of immature neutrophils).

(3) Imaging characteristics. Radiographic examination revealing patchy infiltrates, lobular/segmental consolidation, or interstitial changes with or without pleural effusion.

If any items in (2) is positive and the imaging results support, a diagnosis of community-acquired pneumonia could be made after ruling out non-infectious diseases.

16. Which pathogens cause community-acquired pneumonia?

The most common pathogens that cause acute respiratory diseases include bacteria, viruses, or a combination of bacteria and virus. New pathogens, such as the novel coronavirus, can cause an epidemic or pandemic of an acute respiratory disease.

Bacteria are the main cause of community-acquired pneumonia. Streptococcus pneumonia is one of the most common bacterial pneumonia. Other bacterial pathogens include Mycoplasma, Chlamydia, Klebsiella pneumoniae, Escherichia coli, and Staphylococcus aureus; pneumonia caused by Pseudomonas aeruginosa and Acinetobacter baumannii have also been reported.

The virus detection rate for adult CAP patients in China is 15% to 34.9%, with influenza viruses including Haemophilus influenzae occupying the top spot. Other viral pathogens include parainfluenza virus, rhinovirus, adenovirus, human metapneumovirus, respiratory syncytial virus, and coronavirus. 5.8% to 65.7% of patients with positive virus test results are coinfected with bacteria or atypical pathogens.

17. How is community-acquired pneumonia transmitted?

Theoretically, all pathogens that cause community-acquired pneumonia have potential for human-to-human transmission. Routes of transmission from the source of infection to susceptible populations are droplet transmission, contact transmission, and airborne transmission.

Apart from the cold weather, the major factors such as movement of population (for example, the sizable migration during Spring Festival in China) makes winter more likely for respiratory infectious diseases to strike. It is mainly transmitted through droplets emitted by the patients or virus carriers when they cough or sneeze.

18. What are the risk factors for transmission of community-acquired pneumonia?

Autumn and winter are seasons prone to see the prevalence of respiratory viruses such as influenza, and various other respiratory infections may occur. This made it difficult to distinguish the early stage of COVID-19 from other upper respiratory infections.

The main sources of infection in community-acquired pneumonia include patients, their families, visitors, and their living environment.

The dissemination and outcomes of community-acquired pneumonia are associated with the following factors.

(1) Environmental conditions: air pollutants, overcrowding in confined spaces, humidity, indoor hygiene, seasons, and temperature.

(2) Accessibility and effectiveness of health care services and infection prevention measures: Accessibility and availability of vaccines and health care facilities, and isolation capabilities.

(3) Host factors: age, smoking habits, transmissibility, immune status, nutritional status, previous infection or co-infection of other pathogens, and overall health.

(4) Pathogen characteristics: routes of transmission, infectivity, virulence, and microbial population (inoculation size).

19. How to prevent community-acquired pneumonia?

Control the source of infection: When coughing or sneezing, the patient with acute respiratory diseases should cover their nose and mouth with the arm or other materials (handkerchiefs, paper towels, or masks) to reduce droplet transmission. After exposure to respiratory secretions, perform hand hygiene immediately, and wash hands frequently in daily life.

Personal precautions are as follows:

(1) Maintain a balanced diet, ensuring adequate nutrition, and maintaining oral health can help prevent against infection.

(2) Exercise regularly to boost immunity.

(3) Quit smoking, limit alcohol consumption, and stay in good spirits.

(4) Ensure indoor ventilation: natural ventilation and/or use of exhaust fans for better airflow.

(5) Get vaccinated if available.

20. Who are susceptible to 2019-nCoV?

The novel coronavirus is newly emergent in humans. Therefore, the general population is susceptible because they lack immunity against it. 2019-nCoV can infect individuals with normal or compromised immunity. The amount of exposure to the virus also determines whether you get infected or not. If you are exposed to a large amount of virus, you may get sick even if your immune function is normal. For people with poor immune function, such as the elderly, pregnant women or people with liver or kidney dysfunction, the disease progresses relatively quickly and the symptoms are more severe.

The dominant factor determining whether one gets infected or not is the chance of exposure. So, it cannot be simply concluded that better immunity will lower one's risk of being infected. Children have fewer chances of exposure and thus a lower probability of infection. However, at the same exposure, senior people, people with chronic diseases or compromised immunity are more likely to get infected.

21. What are the epidemiological characteristics of COVID-19?

The emergent epidemic of COVID-19 has experienced three stages: local outbreak, community communication, and widespread stage (epidemic).

Transmission dynamics: in the early stage of the epidemic, the average incubation period was 5.2 days; the doubling time of the epidemic was 7.4 days, i.e., the number of people infected doubled every 7.4 days; the average continuous interval (the average interval time of transmission from one person to another) was 7.5 days; the basic regeneration index (R0) was estimated to be 2.2-3.8, meaning that each patient infects 2.2-3.8 people on average.

Main average intervals: for mild cases, the average interval from onset to the initial hospital visit was 5.8 days, and that from onset to hospitalization 12.5 days; for severe cases, the average interval from onset to hospitalization was 7 days and that from onset to diagnosis 8 days; for fatality cases, the average interval from onset to diagnosis was significantly longer (9 days), and that from onset to death was 9.5 days.

Communication stages: The COVID-19 epidemic passed three stages: 1) the stage of local outbreak (cases of this stage are mostly related to the exposure of a seafood market); 2) the stage of community communication (interpersonal communication and clustering transmission in communities and families); 3) widespread stage (rapid spread, with large population flow, to the entire country of China and even the world.)

22. What are the routes of transmission of 2019-nCoV?

At present, it is believed that transmission through respiratory droplets and contacts is the main routes, but there is a risk of fecal-oral transmission. Aerosol transmission, mother to child transmission and other routes are not confirmed yet.

(1) Respiratory droplets transmission: This is the main mode of direct contact transmission. The virus is transmitted through the droplets generated when patients are coughing, sneezing or talking, and susceptible persons may get infected after inhalation of the droplets.

(2) Indirect contact transmission: The virus can be transmitted through indirect contacts with an infected person. The droplets containing the virus are deposited on the surface of the object, which may be touched by the hand. The virus from the contaminated hand may get passed to the mucosa (or mucosae) of oral cavity, nose and eyes of the person and lead to infection.

(3) The live novel coronavirus has been detected from feces of confirmed patients, suggesting the possibility of fecal-oral transmission.

(4) Aerosol transmission: When the droplets are suspended in the air and lose water, pathogens left behind to form the core of the droplets (i.e. aerosols). Aerosols can fly to a distance, causing long-distance transmission. This mode of transmission is called aerosol transmission. There is no evidence that the novel coronavirus can be transmitted through aerosol yet.

(5) Mother to child transmission: A child of the mother with COVID-19 was confirmed to have positive throat swabs after 30 hours of birth. This suggests that the novel coronavirus may cause neonatal infection through mother to child transmission, but more scientific researches and evidence are in need to confirm this route.

23. What is droplet transmission?

A droplet generally refers to a water-containing particle with a diameter greater than 5 μm.

Droplets can enter mucosal surfaces within a certain distance (typically 1 m). Due to the relatively large size and weight of the droplets, they cannot stay suspended in the air for too long.

Generation of respiratory droplets:

(1) Coughing, sneezing or talking.

(2) During invasive respiratory tract procedures, such as suctioning or bronchoscopy, tracheal intubation, cough-stimulating movements including changing positions in bed or patting backs, and cardiopulmonary resuscitation, etc.

Pathogens transmitted by droplets: influenza virus, SARS coronavirus, adenovirus, rhinovirus, mycoplasma, group A streptococcus and meningococcus (Neisseria), and recently discovered 2019-nCoV.

24. What is airborne transmission?

Airborne transmission is also known as aerosol transmission. Aerosols are suspensions of tiny particles or droplets that can be transmitted through the air. They are generally considered to be less than 5 μm in diameter, and the pathogens carried by them can still be infectious after traveling long distances. Airborne pathogens can also be transmitted through direct contact. The airborne pathogens are classified as follows.

(1) Through the airborne route only: Mycobacterium tuberculosis, Aspergillus.

(2) Through multiple routes, but mainly airborne: measles virus, varicella-zoster virus.

(3) Usually through other routes, but can also be transmitted through airborne only in special scenarios (like tracheal intubation/incision, open-airway suctioning and other aerosol-generating procedures): smallpox virus, SARS coronavirus, 2019-nCoV, Influenza virus and norovirus etc.

25. What is contact transmission?

Contact transmission refers to the transmission of pathogens through direct or indirect contact through fomites (pathogen-carrying objects).

(1) Direct contact. Pathogens are transmitted through direct mucosal or skin contact with an infected host.
- Blood or bloody fluids enter the body through mucous membranes or non-intact skins (mainly viruses).
- Transmission caused by contact with secretions containing certain pathogens, commonly for infections by bacteria, viruses, parasites etc.

(2) Indirect contact. Pathogens are transmitted through contaminated objects or people. Pathogens of intestinal infectious diseases are mostly transmitted through indirect contact.

(3) Other important pathogens transmitted through indirect contact: MRSA (benzoxazole/methicillin-resistant Staphylococcus aureus), VRE (vancomycin-resistant enterococcus), Clostridium difficile.

26. What is a close contact?

Close contacts refer to persons who have contact with a patient who is confirmed or suspected with infection of 2019-nCoV), including the following situations.

(1) Those who live, study, work or have other forms of a close contact with a patient.

(2) Medical personnel, family members or others who have had a close contact with a patient without taking effective protective measures during diagnosing, treatment, nursing and visiting.

(3) Other patients and their accompanying people sharing the same ward with an infected patient.

(4) Those who shared the same transportation or elevator with the patient.

(5) Those who are deemed as such through on-the-spot investigations.

27. Why should close contacts be put under isolated medical observation for 14 days?

Currently the longest incubation period observed for 2019-nCoV is generally 14 days.

Strict monitoring of close contacts and other preventive measures are necessary. This is not only a socially responsible practice for the public health and safety but also consistent with the international convention. With reference to the incubation periods of diseases caused by other coronaviruses, the information from the recent cases of 2019-nCoV, and the current prevention and control practices, close contacts should be placed under medical observation for 14 days at home.

III. Detection, Diagnosis and Treatment

28. What are the clinical manifestations of COVID-19?

The onset of COVID-19 is mainly manifested as fever, but some early patients may not have fever, with only chills and respiratory symptoms, which can occur together with mild dry cough, fatigue, poor breathing, diarrhea etc. However, runny nose, sputum and other symptoms are rare. Patients may gradually develop dyspnea. In severe cases, the disease can progress rapidly, causing acute respiratory distress syndrome, septic shock, irreversible metabolic acidosis, and coagulation disorders in just a matter of days. Some patients start out with mild symptoms without fever. The majority of patients have a good prognosis, while a few become critically and sometimes fatally ill.

29. Do you know something on laboratory testing for COVID-19?

2019-nCoV can be identified by real-time reverse transcription polymerase chain reaction (rRT-PCR). For each case, specimens to be tested should be from lower respiratory tracts, such as bronchial/alveolar lavage fluid and deep sputum. Also, serum samples should be collected both at the onset of symptoms and after 14 days.

In the early stages of the disease, the white blood cell count stays normal or lower, but the lymphocyte count is decreased. While some patients have elevated liver enzymes, muscle enzymes, and myoglobin, most patients have elevated C-reactive protein and erythrocyte sedimentation rate. The procalcitonin levels stay normal and D-dimer is elevated in severe cases.

30. What are the characteristics of COVID-19 chest films?

In the early stages, chest films feature multiple small patchy shadows and interstitial changes, especially in the peripheral third of the chest, which then progress to bilateral ground glass opacities and pulmonary infiltrates. In severe cases, pulmonary consolidations and even "white-out" of the lungs are seen. Pleural effusions are rare.

31. How to identify COVID-19 cases clinically?

Persons who meet both the following conditions are considered suspected cases.

1) Epidemiological history. The case has a travel or residence history in the epidemic areas within two weeks of the onset, or had a contact(s) with patients from the epidemic areas within 14 days of the onset, or other patients with fever and respiratory symptoms in the communities with reported cases or clustered outbreak.

(2) Clinical features. The most common symptom is fever. Some patients may not present with fever, but only chills and respiratory symptoms. Chest films show characteristics of viral pneumonia. During the early stage of the disease, white blood cell count is normal or below normal, while lymphocyte count may decrease.

32. How to confirm COVID-19 cases?

Once a case is identified as a suspected case, a positive result for 2019-nCoV nucleic acid on rRT-PCR testing of specimens (sputum, throat swabs, lower respiratory tract secretions etc.) or highly homologous sequences to the known novel coronavirus found after gene sequencing of the virus from a patient can confirm the diagnosis.

33. How to diagnose severe COVID-19 cases?

Severe cases refer to patients with unstable vital signs and rapid disease progression, with dysfunction or even failures of more than two organ systems. The progression of the disease may endanger the lives of patients.

34. What is the difference between COVID-19 and other pneumonia?

(1) Bacterial pneumonia. Common symptoms include coughing, coughing up sputum, or exacerbation of the original respiratory symptoms, with purulent or bloody sputum, with or without chest pain. It is generally not considered a contagious disease.

(2) SARS/MERS. Although the novel coronavirus is in the same family as SARS and MERS coronaviruses, a genetic evolution analysis shows that it belongs to a different branch of the same subgroup. It is neither a SARS nor a MERS virus, based on the viral genomic sequences. Due to the similarities between COVID-19- and SARS/MERS-caused pneumonia, it is challenging to distinguish them with clinical manifestations and imaging results. Therefore, a pathogen identification test by rRT-PCR is needed.

(3) Other viral pneumonia. Pneumonia caused by influenza virus, rhinovirus, adenovirus, human metapneumovirus, respiratory syncytial virus and other coronaviruses.

35. What should close contacts do with notice from Center of Disease Control?

Please follow the self-monitoring instructions and stay at home. Don't panic. Don't go to work. Don't go out too often. Perform daily checks of health condition and report the records to the authority, and follow up with your community doctors regularly. If fever, cough or other symptoms appear, please go to community health centers for further evaluation and treatment.

36. What should I do if I am possibly infected with COVID-19?

Promptly go to the local designated medical institution for evaluation, diagnosis and treatment. When a seeking medical attention for a possible infection of 2019-nCoV, you should inform your doctor about your recent travel and residence history, especially if you've been to the epidemic areas recently, and any history of contact with pneumonia patients or suspected 2019-nCoV cases, and animals. It is extra important to note that surgical masks should be worn throughout the visit to protect yourself and others.

37. How to choose a medical institution for treatment?

Isolation and treatment should be performed in a hospital with proper conditions for isolation and protection. Critical cases should be admitted to an ICU as soon as possible.

38. What should be done if a patient requires transportation?

Patients should be transported in designated vehicles that are regularly disinfected and manned with well protected personnel.

39. Are there any drugs or vaccines against COVID-19?

At present, there are no specific antiviral treatments against COVID-19. Patients generally receive supportive care to relieve symptoms. Avoid irresponsible or inappropriate antimicrobial treatment, especially in combination with broad-spectrum antimicrobials.

There is currently no vaccine against the new disease. Developing a new vaccine may take a while.

40. How to treat COVID-19?

(1) Put patients to bed rest, provide with supportive care, maintain good hydration and electrolyte balance, internal homeostatis, and closely monitor vital signs and oxygen saturation.

(2) Monitor routine blood and urine test results, C-reactive protein (CRP), biochemical indicators (liver enzyme, myocardial enzyme, renal function, etc.), and coagulation function accordingly. Perform an arterial blood gas analysis when needed, and regularly review chest X-ray images.

(3) According to the changes in oxygen saturation, provide a timely effective oxygen therapy, including nasal catheter, oxygen mask, transnasal high-flow oxygen therapy, and noninvasive or invasive mechanical ventilation, etc.

(4) Antiviral therapy: There are currently no antiviral drugs with good efficacy.

(5) Apply antibacterial drug treatment: strengthen bacteriological monitoring, and start antibacterial treatment when there is evidence of secondary bacterial infection.

(6) Traditional Chinese medicine treatment. Treat according to the syndrome.

41. What are the clinical criteria for quarantine release and discharge?

(1) The condition of the patient is stable and fever has subsided.

(2) Lung imaging shows a significant improvement with no sign of organ dysfunction.

(3) The patient has had stable breathing, clear consciousness, unimpaired speech, normal diet and body temperature for more than 3 days. Respiratory symptoms have improved significantly, and two consecutive tests for respiratory pathogenic nucleic acid have been negative (at least one day in-between tests).

IV. Personal Precautions

42. How to prevent respiratory infections in spring and winter?

Wash hands frequently with plain or antimicrobial soap and rinse with running water. Be sure to dry hands with clean towels. Wash hands immediately after contact with respiratory secretions (for example after sneezing).

Practice good respiratory hygiene/cough practices. Cover mouth and nose while coughing/sneezing with tissue, towel etc. and avoid touching eyes, nose or mouth afterwards before thoroughly washing hands.

Strengthen overall health and immunity. Keep a balanced diet, get enough sleep and regular exercise, and also avoid overworking.

Maintain good hygiene and proper ventilation. Open windows regularly throughout the day to let in fresh air.

Avoid crowded places or contact with persons with respiratory infections.

Seek a medical attention if fever, cough, sneezing, runny nose or other respiratory symptoms appear.

43. Why does flu caused by viruses become pandemic?

Influenza is mainly transmitted through respiratory droplets and contact from infected to susceptible people, or through contact with contaminated items. In general, its incidence peaks in autumn and winter. Human influenza is mainly caused by influenza A virus and influenza B virus. Influenza A viruses often undergo antigen mutations and can be further classified into subtypes such as H1N1, H3N2, H5N1, and H7N9. When new influenza virus subtypes appear, they easily become a pandemic because the population generally lacks immunity against them.

44. How to keep yourself away from the novel coronavirus?

(1) 2019-nCoV is mainly transmitted by droplets and contacts, therefore medical surgical masks must be worn properly.

(2) When sneezing or coughing, do not cover nose and mouth with bare hands but use a tissue or a mask instead.

(3) Wash hands properly and frequently. Even if there are viruses present on hands, washing hands can block the viruses from entering respiratory tract through nose or mouth.

(4) Boost your immunity, and avoid going to crowded and enclosed places. Exercise more and have a regular sleep schedule. Boosting your immunity is the most important way to avoid being infected.

(5) Be sure to wear the mask always! Just in case you come in contact with an infected person, wearing a mask can prevent you from inhaling virus-carrying droplets directly.

45. Can a mask block such small coronaviruses?

The masks are effective. Because the purpose of wearing the mask is to block the 'carrier' by which the virus is transmitted, rather than directly blocking the viruses. Common routes for transmission of respiratory viruses include close contact over a short distance and aerosol transmission over a long distance. Aerosols which people usually come in contact with refer to respiratory droplets from patients. Wearing a mask properly can effectively block respiratory droplets and therefore prevent the virus from directly entering the body.

Please be reminded that it is not necessary to wear a KN95 or N95 respirator. Regular surgical masks can block most virus-carrying droplets from entering the respiratory tract.

46. What are the features of masks for different purposes?

Major types of masks: N95/KN95 respirators, surgical face masks, and cotton face masks.

N95/KN95 respirators can filter 95% of particles with an aerodynamic diameter greater than or equal to 0.3 µm, and block viruses. They can help prevent airborne diseases.

Disposable surgical face masks have 3 layers. The outer layer is hydrophobic non-woven layer which prevents droplets from entering the mask; the middle layer has a filter to block 90% of particles with a diameter greater than 5µm; and the inner layer in contact with the nose and mouth absorbs moisture. They are typically for sterile medical operations and be used to prevent airborne diseases.

Cotton face masks are heavy, stuffy, and do not fit closely to the face, and thus not effective against viruses.

The characteristics of the commonly-used masks are shown in the table on page 24.

47. Any difference between KN95 respirator and N95 respirator?

Respirators are a kind of respiratory protective gear. It's designed to more closely fit on the face than regular masks, and effectively filter particles in the air. "N" indicates "non-oil-based uses" and a N95 mask can be used to protect against non-oil-based suspended particles; "95" means that the filtration efficiency is no less than 95%, indicating that this respirator, as proved by careful testing, can block at least 95% of very small (0.3 µm in size) tested particles.

If worn correctly, N95's filtration efficiency is superior to regular and surgical masks. However, even if you wear it as required, it does not 100% eliminate the risks of infection.

KN95 is one of the ratings specified in the Chinese standard (GB 2626—2006) while N95 is one of the ratings specified in the American standard (42 CFR 84). The technical requirements and testing methods of these two ratings are basically the same, and they both have a filtration efficiency of 95% by their respective standards.

MASK TYPES	INTENDED USE	FILTRATION EFFICIENCY	NUMBER OF USES
N95 masks (Without a breathing valve)	Also known as N95 respirators. A type of respiratory protective gear that can effectively filter particulates in the air and is suitable for protecting against airborne respiratory infectious diseases.	Blocks at least 95% of very small particles (approximately 0.3 µm in size)	Can be reused or used extendedly. Discard the masks when they get damaged, deformed, wet or dirty.
N95 masks (With a breathing valve)	Same as N95 masks without a breathing valve. The breathing valve has a delicate design with several flaps. It allows the exhaled air to escape without letting small particles enter. This design makes exhaling easier and helps reduce the accumulation of moisture and heat.	Same as N95 masks without an exhalation valve. It blocks at least 95% of very small particles (approximately 0.3 µm in size)	Same as N95 masks without a breathing valve.
Surgical masks	Used as basic protective gear for medical professionals or related personnel. It protects the wearer from splashes and droplets that may contain germs.	The filtration efficiency of surgical masks is not uniform. Some might perform worse than required of surgical masks or medical protective masks. In general, particles that are roughly 5 µm in size can be filtered out. There is a water-repelling outer layer which blocks droplets from entering the mask; the middle layer is a filter layer.	Single use
General medical masks	Single-use protection masks for medical procedures. Generally used in ordinary environments to block particles (such as pollen) other than pathogenic microorganisms.	Does not fulfill the filtration efficiency requirements for particles and bacteria, or has lower requirements than surgical masks and medical protective masks.	Single use
Cotton face masks	Used to keep warm and block larger particles such as dust.	Can only filter larger particles, such as soot or dust.	Washable and reusable

48. How to choose a mask?

The capability of masks to protect a wearer is ranked as follows: N95 respirators > surgical face masks > general medical masks > cotton masks.

N95 respirators come in two types, with or without breathing valves. While N95 respirators may make breathing more difficult for people with chronic respiratory diseases, heart disease, or other diseases with breathing difficulty, N95 respirators with breathing valves can make breathing easier and help reduce heat build-up.

N95 respirators with or without breathing valves have the same protection capability for the wearer. However, N95 respirators with breathing valves cannot protect people nearby an infected wearer. Therefore, carriers of the virus should wear N95 respirators without breathing valves to prevent spreading the virus. To keep the sterility of an environment, N95 respirators with breathing valves are not suggested because the wearer may exhale bacteria or viruses.

49. How to put on, use and take off a mask?

(1) After identifying the front, back, top, and bottom of the mask, wash your hands before wearing it. Make sure that the mask covers your nose and mouth, fits closely around the face to form a closed environment, so air passes through the mask, but not the gaps around it. Then, place the ear loops around each the ears.

(2) Besides the front and back side, the surgical mask also has a stiff bendable strip on top. When wearing it, with the front side facing outwards, you also need to make sure the stiff bendable strip is on top, molded around the nose.

(3) Wash hands thoroughly before taking off your mask. Push the front side of mask with one hand while holding the ear loops and remove them from around each ear with the other. Fold the mask with the back side in. If the back side is not contaminated, a limited reuse is allowed.

50. How often should a mask be replaced? Can N95 respirators be extendedly used or reused?

All masks have a limited protective effect and need to be re-placed regularly in the following cases:
- when it is difficult to breath though the mask;
- when the mask is damaged;
- when the mask cannot fit snugly to the contour of the face;
- when the mask is contaminated with blood or respiratory droplets etc.;
- after contact with, or exit from, an isolation ward of any pa-tient infected with an infectious disease requiring contact precautions (the mask has been contaminated).

At present, international organizations including the World Health Organization, have no definitive guidelines as to the opti-mal wearing time of N95 respirators. China has not yet introduced the relevant guidelines regarding the time of use of masks, ei-ther. Researches on the protective capability and wearing time of N95 respirators show that the filtration capability stays at 95% or above after 2 days of use, while the respiratory impedance has not changed much; the filtration capability is reduced to 94.7% after 3 days of use. The U.S. Centers for Disease Control and Prevention recommends that when N95 respirators are in short supply, N95 respirators can be extendedly used or reused unless they are visi-bly dirty or damaged (such as creased or torn).

51. How to keep my glasses from fogging up with a mask on?

To prevent glasses from fogging up while wearing a mask, please wash your hands before touching the mask, make sure the mask is worn in a correct orientation, make sure it fits your face snugly to form a closed environment allowing air to pass through the mask instead of the gaps around it.

52. How should special populations choose a mask?

(1) Pregnant women should choose masks they find comfortable for them. It is suggested that pregnant women consult with doctors for professional instructions on wearing masks.

(2) The elderly and patients with chronic diseases should ask for professional instructions on wearing masks because the body conditions of these people vary. For example, patients with heart and lung diseases may feel uncomfortable when wearing a mask, and it may even aggravate their illnesses.

(3) Generally, children's face is small, so it is recommended that children wear masks specially made for the underaged by reputable manufacturers.

53. Why is handwashing important in preventing respiratory diseases?

The hands are the key medium in transmission of viruses that are transmitted through water, food, blood or blood products, respiratory droplets, digestive tract, in addition to direct or indirect touching. Studies show that proper handwashing is one of the most effective measures to prevent diarrhea and respiratory infections.

54. How to wash hands correctly?

Step 1: Apply soap to hands and scrub palm to palm with fingers interlaced.

Step 2: Put one palm on the back of another hand and scrub your fingers. Change hands.

Step 3: Scrub between your fingers.

Step 4: Rub the back of your fingers against your palms. Do the same with the other hand.

Step 5: Scrub your thumb using the other hand. Do the same with the other thumb.

Step 6: Rub the tips of your fingers on the palm of the other hand

Step 7: Rub the wrist of one hand with the other hand while rotating it. Do the same with the other hand.

In each of the above steps, do each step no fewer than 5 times, and finally rinse your hands under running water.

55. What are the key moments for hand hygiene in daily life?

(1) When you cover a cough or a sneeze with your hand.
(2) After caring for a patient.
(3) Before, during, and after preparing food.
(4) Before eating.
(5) After going to the toilet.
(6) After touching animals.
(7) After touching elevator buttons and door handles or knobs.
(8) After coming home from outside.

56. How to clean hands if clean water is not available?

You can clean your hands with an alcohol-based hand sanitizer. Coronaviruses are not resistant to acid or alkali but are sensitive to organic solvents and disinfectants. 75% alcohol can inactivate the virus, so alcohol-containing disinfection products of an absolute (100%) concentration can be used as an alternative to washing hands with soap and running water.

57. Does handwashing with soap and clean water work against coronaviruses?

Yes, it does. Frequent hand washing is one of the effective measures to prevent viral infection such as rhinovirus and coronavirus. Rubbing hands with soap and water can effectively remove dirt and microorganisms on the skin, and rinsing out the soap under running water can also relieve irritation to the skin. Therefore, authoritative organizations such as the Chinese Center for Disease Control and Prevention, the World Health Organization, and the United States Centers for Disease Control and Prevention all recommend washing hands thoroughly with soap and running water.

58. Can 75% alcohol reduce risk of 2019-nCoV infection?

Yes. Coronaviruses are sensitive to organic solvents and disinfectants. 75% alcohol, chloroform, formaldehyde, chlorine-containing disinfectants, peracetic acid, and ultraviolet rays can inactivate the virus, so wiping hands and mobile phones with alcohol can prevent COVID-19 infection.

59. How to take care of the COVID-19 patient at home?

(1) Quarantine the patient from the rest of the family members and maintain a distance of at least one meter.

(2) Wear a mask when looking after the patient. Discard the mask after each use.

(3) Wash hands thoroughly with soap after having contact with the patient. The patient's living space should be well ventilated.

60. Is it necessary for suspected cases with mild symptoms to be quarantined at home?

Yes. In case of insufficient treatment capacity and medical resources, The World Health Organization recommends that patients with mild symptoms (low-grade fever, coughing, sneezing, and asymptomatic sore throat) and no chronic diseases (such as lung diseases, heart diseases, kidney failure, or immune diseases) could be quarantined at home.

Notes:

(1) During the quarantine at home, patient needs to keep in touch with medical professionals until a full recovery.

(2) Medical professionals must monitor the development of symptoms to assess the patient's condition.

(3) Patients and family members should maintain good hygiene and receive health care, prevention instructions and monitoring.

Caution! Deciding whether a patient is to receive home quarantine requires careful clinical assessment of safety and health risks involved in home healthcare.

61. How to home quarantine for suspected infections?

(1) Arrange a well-ventilated single room for the patient.

(2) Limit the number of caretakers. It is better to designate one person who is in good health and has no chronic diseases to take care of the patient. All visits should be avoided.

(3) Family members of the patient should live in different rooms or at least keep more than one meter from the patient. Nursing mothers can continue to breastfeed their babies.

(4) Restrict the movement of the patient and minimize the shared areas between the patient and family members. Make sure that the shared areas (kitchen, bathroom, etc.) are well-ventilated by opening windows frequently.

(5) Wear a mask when staying in the same room with the patient. The mask should fit the face snugly. Avoid touching or adjusting the mask with unclean hands. Replace the mask immediately when it is contaminated. Wash hands after removing the mask.

(6) Wash hands after having any direct contact with the patient, or entering or exiting the patient's isolation ward. Wash hands before and after preparing food, before eating, after going to the toilet, and when hands look dirty. If hands are not visibly dirty, clean them with a hand sanitizer; if hands are visibly dirty, wash them with soap and water.

(7) After washing hands with soap and water, it is best to use disposable paper towels to dry hands. If they are not available, wipe them with a clean and dry textile towel, and replace it when it becomes wet.

(8) Maintain good hygiene of the respiratory tract (wear masks, use tissues or lift your elbow to cover your mouth when coughing or sneezing, and wash hands immediately after coughing and sneezing).

(9) Disinfect and discard the items used to cover the nose and mouth, or wash them properly after use (such as washing handkerchiefs with soap or detergent and water).

(10) Avoid direct contact with human droplets, especially oral or respiratory secretions, and avoid direct contact with patient's stool.

(11) Wear single-use gloves when cleaning the mouth and respiratory tract of patients as well as handling the patient's feces and urine. Do not discard the gloves carelessly.

(12) Avoid direct contact with the patient or items contaminated by the patient, such as toothbrushes, tableware, food, drinks, towels, bath towels, bed sheets, etc. Wash dishes with detergent or discard them after use.

(13) Use ordinary household disinfectants containing diluted bleach (bleach: water = 1: 99) (most household bleaches contain 5% sodium hypochlorite) to regularly clean and disinfect the frequently-touched objects, such as bedside tables, bed frame and another bedroom furniture. Clean and disinfect bathroom and toilet surfaces at least once a day.

(14) Use ordinary laundry detergent and water to wash the patient's clothing, bed sheets, bath towels, towels, etc., or wash them in a washing machine at 140-194°F with ordinary household laundry detergent, and then dry the above items completely. Put contaminated bedding in laundry bags. Do not shake contaminated clothing to avoid direct contact with skin and your clothes.

(15) Wear disposable gloves and protective clothing (such as a plastic apron) before cleaning and touching clothing, bedding and surfaces of objects contaminated by human secretions. Wash hands before putting on gloves and after removing them.

(16) Patients should stay at home until a full recovery. Deciding whether the patient has recovered requires clinical and/or laboratory diagnosis (rRT-PCR assays should be carried out at least two times and produce negative results; the interval between two consecutive assays should be at least 24 hours).

62. What should I do amid a close contact with a COVID-19 patient?

Monitoring close contacts: All persons (including medical professionals) who may have been in contact with a suspected case should have a 14-day medical observation. The observation starts from the last day of contact with the patient. Seek medical help as soon as you experience any symptoms, especially fever, respiratory symptoms such as coughing, shortness of breath, or diarrhea. During the observation, contacts should keep in touch with medical professionals.

Medical professionals should inform the contacts in advance, if symptoms present, where they can seek medical help, the most suggested transportation, when and where to enter a designated hospital, and what infection control measures to take. Specific instructions are as follows:

(1) Notify the hospital in advance and inform them that a contact with symptoms is going to the hospital.

(2) Wear a surgical mask on the way to the hospital.

(3) Avoid taking public transportation to the hospital. Call an ambulance or use a private vehicle, and try to keep the windows open on the road.

(4) Close contacts of patients should maintain respiratory hygiene at all time and wash their hands frequently. Stay far away from other people (> 1 m) while standing or sitting on the road to or at the hospital.

(5) Contacts of patients and their caregivers should wash their hands properly.

(6) Any surfaces contaminated with respiratory secretions or bodily fluids on the way to the hospital should be cleaned and disinfected with ordinary household disinfectants containing diluted bleach.

63. How to control hospital infection?

The medical workers must strictly follow hygiene and infection control standards in healthcare facilities and the medical procedure protocols to reduce the transmission risks. They must take a better control of hospital infection by practicing good personal protection measures, hand hygiene, ward management, environmental disinfection and waste management.

Pre-examination and triage office/station: wear protective work clothes, work caps, medical surgical masks, etc.

Outpatient, emergency, fever outpatient and isolation ward: during daily consultations and rounds, wear protective work clothes, work caps, medical surgical masks, etc.; when contacting blood, body fluids, secretions or excreta, wear latex gloves; when performing operations/procedures that may incur aerosol or body fluid splashing such as tracheal intubation, airway care and sputum suction, wear N95 masks, facial screens, latex gloves, impermeable isolation clothing, protective clothing and respirator if necessary. The visitation control system should be strictly implemented for the patients in isolation. If it is necessary to visit a patient, the visiting personnel should be instructed for proper personal protection measures according to the relevant regulations.

64. Why do the medical staff of fever clinic wear protective clothing in consultations?

(1) Medical personnel are the main force of epidemic prevention and control. Only when they do well in personal protection can they help patients better.

(2) In order to ensure the health and occupational safety of medical workers so that they can detect and rescue suspected cases in time and effectively, the prevention and control measures and nosocomial infection control must be enhanced in all levels of hospitals, and the protection of medical workers should be strengthened by monitoring their health and providing care and support.

65. What personal protective equipment is required for healthcare institutions?

Medical institutions should be equipped with disposable working caps, disposable surgical face masks, goggles, work clothes (white gown), protective clothing, disposable latex gloves, disposable shoe covers and comprehensive respiratory protective devices or positive pressure headgears, etc.

66. What lifestyle is recommended amid the outbreak of COVID-19?

(1) Eat high-protein foods daily including fish, meat, eggs, milk,

legumes and nuts, keep an adequate intake based on daily diet . Do not eat wild animal meats.

(2) Eat fresh fruits and vegetables every day, and increase the intake based on daily diet.

(3) Drink no less than 1500 mL of water per day.

(4) Have a varied, diverse diet of different types, colors and sources. Eat more than 20 kinds of food every day. Eat a balanced diet of animal- and plant-based foods.

(5) Ensure enough intake of nutrition based on the regular diet.

(6) Undernourished, elderly people and patients with chronic wasting diseases are recommended to supplement with commercial enteral nutrition solutions (foods for special medical purpose), and supplement no less than an extra 2100 kJ daily (500 kcal).

(7) Do not fast or go on a diet during an epidemic of COVID-19.

(8) Ensure regular rest and a minimum of 7 hours of sleep each day.

(9) Start a personal exercise regimen with no less than 1 hour of exercise per day. Do not participate in group exercises.

(10) During an epidemic of COVID-19, it is recommended to supplement with multi-vitamins, minerals, and deep-sea fish oil.

67. How to exercise amid outbreak of COVID-19?

Follow a comprehensive exercise program, increase the intensity progressively, and exercise consistently.

Follow comprehensive exercise programs, exercising every part and system of the body, and expanding the scope and types of your exercise to ensure different attributes of your physical fitness are enhanced.

Increase the intensity progressively. Start exercises from low intensity and gradually scale it up after your body has adapted to the initial intensity. It is suggested to do basic movements and learn easy techniques before moving onto higher level.

(3) Exercise consistently. Keep exercising until it becomes a habit.

68. How do smoking and drinking affect your immune system?

Smoking causes an increase in nicotine concentration in blood, which could result in vasospasm and transient hypoxia in organs. Particularly, the decrease of oxygen in respiratory tract and viscera could damage immunity. Excessive drinking could harm the gastro-intestinal tract, liver, and brain cells, and undermine immunity. It is recommended to quit smoking and limit alcohol intake.

69. How to prevent the infection by the novel coronavirus at home?

(1) Raise health and hygiene awareness. Moderate exercises as well as enough and regular rest can boost immunity.

(2) Maintain good personal hygiene. Cover your nose and mouth with a tissue when coughing or sneezing. Wash hands frequently and avoid touching your eyes, nose, or mouth with unwashed hands.

(3) Maintain good hygiene in rooms, clean floor and furniture, separate household wastes and take out the rubbish timely.

(4) Keep good ventilation. Ventilate every day to let fresh air in.

(5) Disinfection. Apply disinfectant regularly to, and mop the floor and wipe the surface of furniture. The novel coronavirus is sensitive to ultraviolet rays and heat. Sustained heat at 132.8°F for 30 minutes, 75% alcohol, chlorine-containing disinfectants, hydrogen peroxide disinfectants and chloroform can effectively inactivate the virus.

(6) Avoid close contact with people who have symptoms of respiratory diseases (such as fever, cough, sneezing, etc.).

(7) Avoid going to crowded and confined spaces. Wear a mask if you must go.

(8) Do not eat wild animals. Avoid contact with poultry and wild animals, and do not handle fresh meat of wild animals.

(9) Keep pets in strict captivity. Have your pets vaccinated. Maintain good hygiene for pets.

(10) Follow the food safety precautions and habits. Eat thoroughly-cooked meat and hard-boiled eggs.

(11) Pay attention to your body conditions. Seek medical help immediately in cases of symptoms such as fever, cough, etc.

70. How to ventilate my rooms?

The doors and windows of the home are closed most of the time in cold weather, so the air in rooms could be polluted quickly considering the confinement and indoor activities such as cooking. Therefore, windows should be opened from time to time to let fresh air in.

At present, there are no explicit international guidelines for proper ventilation. It is recommended to ventilate according to the environmental conditions indoors and outdoors. Ventilations in the morning, afternoon and evening are suggested when the air outside is good. The ventilation should be kept for 15 to 30 minutes. The frequency and time of ventilation should be decreased accordingly when the outdoor air is in poor quality.

71. How to prevent the infection by 2019-nCoV during travel?

(1) Take a note of the weather at your destination, and bring enough clothes accordingly to keep warm.

(2) Wear a mask while traveling by bus, train or plane, and drink enough water.

(3) Maintain a regular rest schedule during the trip, eat balanced diets and exercise to maintain immunity.

(4) Avoid a long stay in crowded places and wear masks.

(5) Use disposable items to avoid cross infection when receiving guests or going to public places. For example, prepare disposable slippers when having guests at home; use disposable cups; bring your own towels when going to public bathrooms, etc.

(6) Avoid contact with wild animals, stray cats and dogs.

(7) Eat thoroughly-cooked meat because high temperatures can effectively kill viruses in food.

(8) Seek medical help immediately if you have any symptoms of illnesses, and do not travel if you are sick.

72. Which commonly-used Chinese herbs can prevent COVID-19?

Based on the clinical characteristics of COVID-19, it can be classified as an "epidemic" or "pestilent" disease in traditional Chinese medicine. Its core pathogenic factors are "dampness, toxin, stasis and blockage." It mainly affects the lung and spleen, and may injure the collaterals and enter the blood. Drawing upon the clinical experiences of doctors currently treating COVID-19, both national and regional health administrative authorities have recommended specific TCM herbal formulas for treatments. The most commonly used TCM ingredients include: rhizoma phragmitis (lu gen), rhizoma imperatae (bai mao gen), radix angelicae dahuricae (bai zhi), rhizoma atractylodis macrocephalae (bai zhu), rhizoma atractylodis (cang zhu), honeysuckle (jin yin hua), herba pogostemonis (huo xiang), radix et rhizoma rhodiolae crenulatae (hong jing tian), rhizoma dryopteridis crassirhizomatis (guan zhong), rhizoma polygoni cuspidati (hu zhang), fructus tsaoko (cao guo), pericarpium citri reticulatae (chen pi), folium mori (sang ye), radix astragali praeparata (huang qi), radix ligustici brachylobi (fang feng), and herba eupatorii (pei lan). However, it is important to note that herbal formulas should only be used under the guidance of professionally-trained Chinese medicine physicians.

Also note that taking Isatis root (ban lan gen) or fumigating indoor spaces with burning vinegar are not effective means of preventing 2019-nCoV infection.

73. How to get mentally prepared during the outbreak of COVID-19?

(1) Adjust your attitudes and view COVID-19 from a scientific perspective. During the early days of the outbreak, limited knowledge on the risks and prevention of COVID-19 might cause a sense of anxiety and panic among the public, which was exacerbated by rumors. Have confidence in the authoritative efforts for prevention and control and trust scientific research findings of the disease. Adjust your attitudes, act with caution and stay away from fear.

(2) Acknowledge your anxiety and fear. Faced with an unknown epidemic, few people can stay calm. The increased number of confirmed cases would lead to the assumption that the new virus is present everywhere and is unpreventable, causing anxiety and fear. That is natural. Accept the status and avoid excessive self-blame for feeling such emotions.

(3) Maintain a regular and healthy lifestyle: adequate sleep, a healthy balanced diet of diverse food groups, a regular work routine which may help distract ourselves from the epidemic, and a moderate exercise regimen.

(4) Allow yourself to let off steam when you feel necessary. Occasional laughing, crying, shouting, exercising, singing, speaking, chatting, writing, or drawing can help release anger and anxiety, divert your attention, and calm down effectively. Watching TV or listening to music at home also helps to ease anxiety.

(5) Relax and cope with your emotions. Relaxation techniques can help you release your negative emotions such as tension, depression, and anxiety. There are many ways of relaxation and the key to successful relaxation is to understand the basic principles of the techniques and practice.

- Relaxation through visualization. Maintain a slow, steady and deep breath during the whole process, and feel warm energy flowing through your body with visualization.
- Muscle relaxation. Relax your arms, head, trunk and legs successively. Keep the environment quiet, dim the light and minimize sensory stimuli. A simple five-step relaxation cycle consists of: focusing your attention → tensing your muscles → maintaining the tension → releasing the tension → relaxing your muscles.
- Relaxation through deep breathing: this is the easiest way to relax that can be used in any situation where you feel nervous. Steps: stand up straight, put your shoulders down naturally, slightly close your eyes, and then inhale deeply and exhale slowly. It usually takes just a few minutes to feel relaxed.

(6) Seek professional support. Seek counselling or medical treatment for unresolved tension, anxiety, fear, anger, sleep disorder, physical reactions, etc. On a different note, when a quarantined or suspected patient manifests extreme emotions and behaviors, prevention and control professionals should consider the possible onset of psychiatric disorders, and send the person in case to mental health institutions and personnel. Such extreme emotions and behaviors include: anxiety, depression, delusion, restlessness, uncontrollable and improper speech or actions, or even violent refusal or evasion of quarantine, and suicidal ideation.

V. Precautions in Public Places

74. How to prevent infection by 2019-nCoV at farmer's markets?

(1) Avoid contact with livestock or wild animals without protective measures.

(2) Avoid large crowds; wear a mask if contact is unavoidable.

(3) Cough or sneeze into paper tissues, your sleeves or elbows while completely covering the nose and mouth. Seal used tissues in a plastic bag before discarding immediately in a closed bin labeled "residual waste" or "medical waste" to prevent the virus from spreading. After coughing or sneezing, wash hands with soap and water or an alcohol-based hand sanitizer.

(4) Wash hands immediately after returning home. Fever and other symptoms of respiratory infections, especially persistent fever, indicate the need for an immediate hospital visit.

75. How to prevent infection by 2019-nCoV in cinemas and theaters?

During an epidemic outbreak, try to avoid visits to public spaces, especially places with large crowds and poor ventilation like cinemas. Wear a face mask if visits to public spaces are required. Cough or sneeze into tissues completely covering the nose and mouth. Seal used tissues in a plastic bag before discarding immediately in a closed bin labeled "residual waste" or "medical waste" to prevent the virus from spreading. Operators of public spaces should maintain a hygienic indoor environment, ensure regular ventilation and sterilization every day.

76. How to prevent infection by 2019-nCoV when traveling by public transportation?

Passengers on public transport such as bus, metro, ferry or airliners must wear face masks to reduce the risk of getting infected in crowded spaces. Seal used tissues in a plastic bag before discarding immediately in a closed bin labeled "residual waste" or "medical waste" to prevent the virus from spreading.

77. How to prevent infection by 2019-nCoV in the workplace?

Keep the workplace well-ventilated. Do not spit in public; you can spit into a tissue paper and then dispose of it in a closeable bin when convenient. Cough or sneeze into tissues while completely covering the nose and mouth. Seal used tissues in a plastic bag before discarding immediately in a closed bin labeled "residual waste" or "medical waste" to prevent the virus from spreading. Wash hands frequently to maintain personal hygiene; avoid all kinds of social gatherings during the epidemic.

78. How to prevent infection by 2019-nCoV in elevators?

During the 2003 SARS outbreak, an incidence of people becoming infected after taking elevators with cases has been reported.

An elevator carries a high risk of transmission due to its confined space. To prevent the spread of 2019-nCoV in elevators, the following measures should be taken:

(1) The elevator should be thoroughly and regularly disinfected several times with ultraviolet irradiation, 75% alcohol or chlorine-containing disinfectants every day.

(2) Minimize the risks of getting infected from sneezing by taking the elevators alone if possible.

(3) Wear a mask before entering the elevator. If someone sneezes in the elevator while you have no masks on, cover your mouth and nose with your sleeves and measures like clothes changing and personal cleaning should be taken right after.

79. How to prevent infection by 2019-nCoV at wet markets?

(1) Wash hands with soap and clean water after touching animals and animal products.

(2) Disinfect equipment and work area at least once a day.

(3) Wear protective suits, gloves and masks, when handling animals and fresh animal products.

(4) Remove protective clothing after work, clean them daily and leave them in the work area.

(5) Keep family members away from unwashed work clothes, shoes, etc.

80. How to prevent infection by 2019-nCoV in hospitals?

(1) Wear a mask during hospital visits, especially visits to fever clinics or respiratory departments.

(2) Avoid close contact with people presenting symptoms of respiratory diseases (such as fever, cough and sneezing).

(3) Maintain good personal hygiene; cover nose and mouth with tissues when coughing or sneezing.

(4) Wash hands with soap or alcohol-based hand sanitizer. Avoid touching eyes, nose, or mouth without washing hands.

(5) Seal the used tissues in a plastic bag before discarding it in a closed bin of "other wastes" or medical wastes.

81. How to prevent infection by 2019-nCoV in colleges and universities?

(1) Avoid gatherings;

(2) Raise awareness. The departments for safety management should train staff, faculty, and students on proper prevention and personal protection.

(3) Ensure rapid quarantine and notification of staff, faculty, and students with symptoms of fever, cough or other symptoms of respiratory infections. Discourage working or studying during sickness.

(4) Ask students to provide details of the travel history and pay close attention to those who have returned from the regions, communities or families with the confirmed cases.

(5) Screen students for symptoms of fever, cough and other symptoms of respiratory infections in the morning and afternoon.

(6) Ensure an adequate supply of disposable masks, disinfectants, disposable gloves, and hand sanitizers.

(7) The campus infirmary and departments for safety management should guide and supervise the cleaning, ventilation, and disinfection of classrooms, dormitories, canteens, libraries, and other public facilities.

82. How to prevent infection by 2019-nCoV in primary and secondary schools as well as nurseries?

(1) Contingency plans and leadership accountability systems for the prevention and control of 2019-nCoV infection should be established, and responsibilities assigned to departments and individuals.

(2) Campus medical staff and department for safety management should give lectures on the prevention and control of infection to staff, faculty and teachers for their understanding and awareness of the virus.

(3) Campus medical staff and faculty should monitor students' health conditions, carry out morning and afternoon inspections, and check students for fever, cough and other symptoms of respiratory infections. Ensure rapid quarantine of students with symptoms and immediate notification of parents and local health departments.

(4) Keep the campus dry and clean, rooms with adequate ventilation, disinfect public places and facilities daily, and equip hand wash sinks with hand sanitizers or soaps.

(5) Reduce group activities. In classrooms, students should sit separately with adequate distance from each other. Arrange the meal times in canteens in successive, alternating batches.

(6) Contact parents for student information on activities outside the school.

83. How can students avoid infection by 2019-nCoV at learning places?

(1) Classrooms. Compared with other learning places, class-rooms are more crowded. Therefore, keep the classroom clean and disinfect it daily. Ventilate the classroom 3 times every day, each time for 20-30 minutes. People inside should keep warm when ventilating the room. Maintain a proper social distance. Wear a mask, wash hands frequently, drink plenty of water, and avoid shouting or eating in the classroom.

(2) Libraries. The library is an important public learning place for both teachers and students. The library staff should wear protective clothes and keep the library well-ventilated, dry, clean, and disinfected daily. Teachers and students should wash and disinfect their hands after borrowing books. They should wear a face mask and avoid rubbing their eyes, nose or mouth with their hands.

(3) Laboratories. Laboratories are important public place at the school. Disposable latex gloves and masks should be worn when studying or doing experiments in a laboratory. After the experiment is completed, laboratory consumables should be properly disposed of while equipment and utensils should be sterilized promptly. The 7 steps of handwashing (See Question 54) should be followed.

84. How can students avoid infection by 2019-nCoV in their living space?

(1) Canteens. Ensure food safety and hygiene, and strengthen inspection on meat products. Before starting work every day, canteen staff should take temperature, put on masks and wash hands. They should also replace masks regularly according to the guidelines. Areas for food processing and dining as well as tableware should be sterilized with ultraviolet light and high heat every day. Canteen toilets should be equipped with faucets, soap and disinfectants for handwashing. Reduce the number of large dining tables, arrange students and teachers to eat in batches, and maintain a proper distance between people in the queue to avoid over-crowding.

(2) Stadiums. Teachers and students are advised to do moderate exercise, which is beneficial for health. High-intensity exercise or contact sports are not recommended, because the former can weaken people's immunity while the latter can potentially spread the virus.

(3) Dormitories. Dormitories should be well-ventilated and clean. Regular disinfection should be carried out if possible. Students should wash hands after entering the dormitory from outside, and change and wash clothes and take shower regularly. Ensure regular and adequate sleep.

85. How to prevent infection by 2019-nCoV in elder-care settings?

(1) Elder-care facilities should implement a closed-off management that restricts outdoor activities of residents, visits of their relatives and friends, and reception of new residents.

(2) Take the travel history of the residents during the epidemic and immediately quarantine close contacts with confirmed patients.

(3) The managing staff should know how to prevent and control the COVID-19 and take a 24-hour shift to respond to emergencies.

(4) Ensure an adequate supply of personal protective equipment such as face masks and hand sanitizers and distribute them to the residents.

(5) Strengthen hygiene measures, including thorough cleaning of the environment, prompt waste disposal, and daily ventilation and disinfection.

(6) Check body temperature and symptoms related to COVID-19 every day. Ensure rapid quarantine of potentially contagious persons and a prompt notification to the health officials.

(7) Provide education on prevention of infection and encourage good hygiene and health habits.

86. How to prevent infection by 2019-nCoV in canteens?

(1) Canteens should encourage dining in batches and at off-peak meal times to reduce interaction between diners. During meals,

one should avoid face-to-face contact or conversation and should shorten meal times. Diners can also take meals out and use personal cutlery to eat alone; should wash hands before eating and, if eating in a canteen, keep the mask on until sitting down to eat.

(2) Canteens should strengthen personal protection for their employees. In addition to regular protective equipment such as uniforms and hats, all cooks in the kitchen and waiters in the hall should wear masks and single-use gloves and should replace them regularly.

(3) Every morning, canteens should take employees' temperature and screen them for symptoms of fever (over 37.3°C), cough, and fatigue. Ensure rapid quarantine and treatment of employees with such symptoms and disinfect the environment and articles that they had contacted with. Workers with diarrhea, hand injury or other diseases that may affect food safety should be transferred away from their post.

VI. Basics of Contagious Diseases

87. What are notifiable and quarantinable contagious diseases?

Notifiable contagious disease refers to any of various communicable health conditions that upon detection are required to be reported to local public health authorities in a timely manner. For these diseases, mandatory disease reporting plays a critical role in helping the authority to prevent and control the spread of disease in populations.

Quarantinable contagious diseases refer to contagious diseases that are highly contagious and have a high fatality rate, such as plague, cholera, and yellow fever.

In accordance with the *Law of the People's Republic of China on the Prevention and Treatment of Contagious Diseases*, China's health authorities have instituted management of quarantinable contagious diseases for COVID-19 based on the current understanding of its etiology, epidemiology and clinical characteristics. Control of ports, customs, and transportation links according to such management could reduce transmission through humans, animals, and articles.

The principle of China towards the control and prevention of contagious diseases are as follows: (1) prevention first, (2) equal emphasis on both prevention and treatment, (3) classified management of different kinds of contagious diseases, and (4) relying on scientific evidence and the concerted efforts of the public.

88. Why has the COVID-19 been classified as a Class B contagious disease while Class A control measures have been taken?

(1) The novel coronavirus pneumonia is not as serious as other class A contagious diseases (plague and cholera) yet. However, because it is a newly discovered disease, with relative substantial public health risk, everyone needs to be vigilant and well protected.

(2) Taking the Class A control measures brings about faster notifications and publicizing; this facilitates the health workers in prevention and control of the disease as well as the public in acquiring the latest information for a better response to the epidemic.

89. What is a "super-spreader"?

A virus in an infected person can mutate or adapt to the conditions of the human body such that it can infect close contacts more easily. Patients carrying such a virus are called super-spreaders.

If the number of people infected by a patient exceeds three, such patient might be considered a super-spreader; if the number of people infected by a patient exceeds ten, such patients are super-spreaders.

Super-spreaders are also known as "King of viral infection" (Du Wang) in Chinese. The second meaning of "King of viral infection" is that the patients infected by these super-spreaders usually exhibit more severe symptoms and many patients may even die. The super-virulence of the virus spread by a super-spreader is the result of an increased infectivity and pathogenicity due to viral mutations.

90. What is the asymptomatic infection?

It refers to an infection where people with infections are asymptomatic and their physical examination findings could be normal. Often, when the pathogens are reproducing and incubating in the patient body, there is no clinical symptoms or abnormal signs. Without laboratory tests, he/she cannot be diagnosed. Persons with asymptomatic infections, including those of 2019-nCoV, are potential spreaders of the pathogen.

91. What is quarantine for medical observation?

According to the *Law of the People's Republic of China on Prevention and Treatment of Contagious Diseases*, close contacts with individuals known or suspected to be infected with the virus should undergo a medical observation or other preventive measures at the designated places.

The key management measures for close contacts include:

(1) Register them for medical observation for seven to fourteen days.

(2) They should avoid unnecessary outdoor activities.

(3) They should be followed up every day by the disease prevention authority to assess and record body temperature and any symptoms related to COVID-19.

92. How to transport critically ill patients with infections?

For critically ill patients confirmed as 2019-nCoV positive, one should call the local emergency for an arrangement of ambulance transportation. The companion of the patients should wear a mask and protective suits for personal protection. Negative pressure ambulances should be used to prevent spreading the virus in the air. At negative pressure relative to the surrounding areas, air in the ambulance can be filtered and purified before emission, thus minimizing cross infection among the medical staff during treatment and transport of patients. Therefore, technically speaking, negative pressure ambulances are currently the most desirable vehicles for transport of patients with infections.

Appendix: Self-Evaluation Form for Medical Observation at Home

Day	Body Temperature	Spirit	Fatigue	Muscle Soreness	Coughing	Diarrhea	Chest Pain	Breathing Difficulties
1								
2								
3								
4								
5								
6								
7								
8								
9								
10								
11								
12								
13								
14								
Overall Rating								

Notes:

For body temperature, please record the actual measured temperature. For other evaluation items (except for spirit), rate 1 to 5 according to the following coding:

1 = extreme uncomfortable/difficult

2 = very uncomfortable/difficult

3 = moderately uncomfortable/difficult

4 = fairly good/easy

5 = normal/very easy

Please consult your doctor if your body temperature is higher than normal on any given day (normal armpit temperature is 96.8 ~ 98.6°F) or any other evaluation items is rated 1 or 2.

Postscript

In 2003, China suffered the ravage of SARS, which began in Guang-dong province and sent shivers through home and abroad. Studies have confirmed that the coronavirus causing SARS (SARS-CoV) originated from bats and was transmitted to humans through Paguma larvata. As the novel coronavirus pneumonia is spreading, there are studies that suggest the genome of the pathogen (2019-nCov) shows more than 85% homology with a coronavirus in bats. Although it is not yet known which wildlife transmits the virus, the evidence so far is enough to confirm that this is another wildlife-induced human epidemic. In fact, the "culprit" of this disease is not wildlife but humans. Humans' wanton destruction of the natural ecology, wildlife hunting, poor hygiene and bad dietary habits have invited the tragedy again and again. We have reason to believe that the occurrence and spread of contagious diseases is the choice made by nature for rebalancing its relationship with humans.

The progress and development of human society should not be threatened by contagious diseases. Here, we call on everyone to respect nature, value science and adopt healthy lifestyles. We have confidence in overcoming the disease and building a balanced and harmonious relation between humans and nature.

Coronavirus Information from the CDC

Information about the Coronavirus from the CDC (Centers for Disease Control and Prevention) is updated regularly at www.cdc.gov/COVID19. The following is a compilation of important summaries and guidelines about the Coronavirus with specific details last updated by the CDC on February 27, 2020.

Coronavirus Disease 2019 (COVID-19) Situation Summary

This is an emerging, rapidly evolving situation and CDC will provide updated information as it becomes available, in addition to updated guidance.
Updated February 27, 2020

Background

CDC is responding to an outbreak of respiratory disease caused by a novel (new) coronavirus that was first detected in Wuhan City, Hubei Province, China and which has now been detected in 50 locations internationally, including cases in the United States. The virus has been named "SARS-CoV-2" and the disease it causes has been named "coronavirus disease 2019" (abbreviated "COVID-19").

On January 30, 2020, the International Health Regulations Emergency Committee of the World Health Organization declared the outbreak a "public health emergency of international concern" (PHEIC). On January 31, 2020, Health and Human Services Secretary Alex M. Azar II declared a public health emergency (PHE) for the United States to aid the nation's healthcare community in responding to COVID-19.

Source and Spread of the Virus

Coronaviruses are a large family of viruses that are common in many different species of animals, including camels, cattle, cats, and bats. Rarely, animal coronaviruses can infect people and then spread between people such as with MERS-CoV, SARS-CoV, and now with this new virus (named SARS-CoV-2).

The SARS-CoV-2 virus is a betacoronavirus, like MERS-CoV and SARS-CoV. All three of these viruses have their origins in bats. The sequences from U.S. patients are similar to the one that China initially posted, suggesting a likely single, recent emergence of this virus from an animal reservoir.

Early on, many of the patients in the COVID-19 outbreak in Wuhan, China had some link to a large seafood and live animal market, suggesting animal-to-person spread. Later, a growing number of patients reportedly did not have exposure to animal markets, indicating person-to-person spread. Person-to-person spread has been reported outside China, including in the United States and other locations. Chinese officials report that sustained person-to-person spread in the community is occurring in China. In addition, other destinations have apparent community spread, meaning some people have been infected who are not sure how or where they became infected. Learn what is known about the spread of newly emerged coronaviruses: https://www.cdc.gov/coronavirus/2019-ncov/about/transmission.html.

Situation in U.S.

Imported cases of COVID-19 in travelers have been detected in the U.S. Person-to-person spread of COVID-19 also has been reported among close contacts of returned travelers from Wuhan. On February 25, CDC confirmed COVID-19 in a person who reportedly did not have relevant travel history or exposure to another known patient with COVID-19 (unknown exposure). At this time, this virus is NOT currently spreading in the community in the United States.

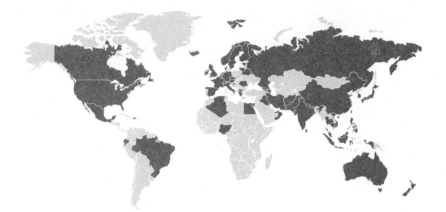

Confirmed COVID-19 Cases Global Map [as of February 27, 2020]

Illness Severity

Both MERS-CoV and SARS-CoV have been known to cause severe illness in people. The complete clinical picture with regard to COVID-19 is not fully understood. Reported illnesses have ranged from mild to severe, including illness resulting in death.

There are ongoing investigations to learn more. This is a rapidly evolving situation and information will be updated as it becomes available.

Risk Assessment

Outbreaks of novel virus infections among people are always of public health concern. The risk from these outbreaks depends on characteristics of the virus, including how well it spreads between people, the severity of resulting illness, and the medical or other measures available to control the impact of the virus (for example, vaccine or treatment medications). The fact that this disease has caused illness, including illness resulting in death, and sustained person-to-person spread is concerning. These factors meet two of the criteria of a pandemic. As community spread is detected in more and more countries, the world moves closer toward meeting the third criteria, worldwide spread of the new virus.

The potential public health threat posed by COVID-19 is high, both globally and to the United States.

But individual risk is dependent on exposure.

- For the general American public, who are unlikely to be exposed to this virus at this time, the immediate health risk from COVID-19 is considered low.
- Under current circumstances, certain people will have an increased risk of infection, for example healthcare workers caring for patients with COVID-19 and other close contacts of persons with COVID-19. CDC has developed guidance to help in the risk assessment and management of people with potential exposures to COVID-19.

However, it's important to note that current global circumstances suggest it is likely that this virus will cause a pandemic. In that case, the risk assessment would be different.

What May Happen

More cases are likely to be identified in the coming days, including more cases in the United States. It's also likely that person-to-person spread will continue to occur, including in the United States. Widespread transmission of COVID-19 in the United States would translate into large numbers of people needing medical care at the same time. Schools, childcare centers, workplaces, and other places for mass gatherings may experience more absenteeism. Public health and healthcare systems may become overloaded, with elevated rates of hospitalizations and deaths. Other critical infrastructure, such as law enforcement, emergency medical services, and transportation industry may also be affected. Health care providers and hospitals may be overwhelmed. At this time, there is no vaccine to protect against COVID-19 and no medications approved to treat it. Nonpharmaceutical interventions would be the most important response strategy.

CDC Response

Global efforts at this time are focused concurrently on containing spread of this virus and mitigating the impact of this virus. The federal government is working closely with state, local, tribal, and territorial partners, as well as public health partners, to respond to this public health threat. The public health response is multi-layered, with the goal of detecting and minimizing introductions of this virus in the United States so as to reduce the spread and the impact of this virus. CDC is operationalizing all of its pandemic preparedness and response plans, working on multiple fronts to meet these goals, including specific measures to prepare communities to respond local transmission of the virus that causes COVID-19. There is an abundance of pandemic guidance developed in anticipation of an influenza pandemic that is being repurposed and adapted for a COVID-19 pandemic.

Highlights of CDC's Response

- CDC established a COVID-19 Incident Management System on January 7, 2020. On January 21, CDC activated its Emergency Operations Center to better provide ongoing support to the COVID-19 response.
- The U.S. government has taken unprecedented steps with respect to **travel** in response to the growing public health threat posed by this new coronavirus:
  - Effective February 2, at 5pm, the U.S. government suspended entry of foreign nationals who have been in China within the past 14 days.
  - U.S. citizens, residents, and their immediate family members who have been in Hubei province and other parts of mainland China are allowed to enter the United States, but they are subject to health monitoring and possible quarantine for up to 14 days.
  - CDC has issued the following travel guidance related to COVID-19:

- China — Level 3, Avoid Nonessential Travel — updated February 22; https://wwwnc.cdc.gov/travel/notices/warning/novel-coronavirus-china
- South Korea — Level 3, Avoid Nonessential Travel — updated February 24; https://wwwnc.cdc.gov/travel/notices/warning/coronavirus-south-korea
- Japan — Level 2, Practice Enhanced Precautions — updated February 22; https://wwwnc.cdc.gov/travel/notices/alert/coronavirus-japan
- Iran — Level 2, Practice Enhanced Precautions — issued February 23; https://wwwnc.cdc.gov/travel/notices/warning/coronavirus-iran
- Italy — Level 2, Practice Enhanced Precautions — issued February 23; https://wwwnc.cdc.gov/travel/notices/warning/coronavirus-italy
- Hong Kong — Level 1, Practice Usual Precautions — issued February 19. https://wwwnc.cdc.gov/travel/notices/watch/coronavirus-hong-kong
- CDC also recommends that all travelers reconsider cruise ship voyages into or within Asia at this time.
- CDC is issuing clinical guidance, including:
  - An interim Health Alert Network (HAN) Update to inform state and local health departments and healthcare professionals about this outbreak on February 1.
  - On January 30, CDC published guidance for healthcare professionals on the clinical care of COVID-19 patients: https://www.cdc.gov/coronavirus/2019-ncov/hcp/clinical-guidance-management-patients.html
  - On February 3, CDC posted guidance for assessing the potential risk for various exposures: https://www.cdc.gov/coronavirus/-2019ncov/php/risk-assessment.html to COVID-19 and managing those people appropriately.
  - On February 27, CDC updated its criteria to guide evaluation of persons under investigation for COVID-19: https://www.cdc.gov/coronavirus/2019-nCoV/hcp/clinical-criteria.html

- CDC has deployed multidisciplinary teams to support state health departments with clinical management, contact tracing, and communications.
- CDC has worked with the Department of State, supporting the safe return of Americans who have been stranded as a result of the ongoing outbreaks of COVID-19 and related travel restrictions. CDC has worked to assess the health of passengers as they return to the United States and provided continued daily monitoring of people who are quarantined.

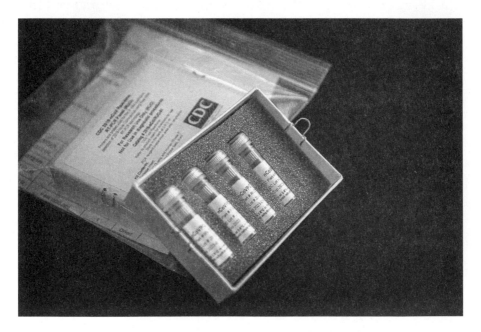

This is a picture of CDC's laboratory test kit for severe acute respiratory syndrome coronavirus 2 (SARS-CoV-2). CDC is shipping the test kits to laboratories CDC has designated as qualified, including U.S. state and local public health laboratories, Department of Defense (DOD) laboratories and select international laboratories. The test kits are bolstering global laboratory capacity for detecting SARS-CoV-2.

- CDC laboratories have supported the COVID-19 response, including:
  - CDC has developed a real time Reverse Transcription-Polymerase Chain Reaction (rRT-PCR) test that can diagnose COVID-19 in respiratory samples from clinical specimens. On January 24, CDC publicly posted the assay protocol for this test: https://www.cdc.gov/coronavirus/2019-nCoV/lab/index.html.
  - On February 26, CDC and FDA developed a protocol that uses two of the three components of the original CDC test kit to detect the virus that causes COVID-19. This will allow at least 40 public health laboratories to be able to begin testing.
  - CDC has been uploading the entire genome of the viruses from reported cases in the United States to GenBank as sequencing was completed.
  - CDC has grown the COVID-19 virus in cell culture, which is necessary for further studies, including for additional genetic characterization. The cell-grown virus was sent to NIH's BEI Resources Repository for use by the broad scientific community.

CDC Recommends

- While the immediate risk of this new virus to the American public is believed to be low at this time, everyone can do their part to help us respond to this emerging public health threat:
  - It's currently flu and respiratory disease season and CDC recommends getting a flu vaccine, taking everyday preventive actions to help stop the spread of germs, and taking flu antivirals if prescribed.
  - If you are a healthcare provider, be on the look-out for people who recently traveled from China and have fever and respiratory symptoms.
  - If you are a healthcare provider caring for a COVID-19

patient or a public health responder, please take care of yourself and follow recommended infection control procedures.

- If you have been in China or have been exposed to someone sick with COVID-19 in the last 14 days, you will face some limitations on your movement and activity. Please follow instructions during this time. Your cooperation is integral to the ongoing public health response to try to slow spread of this virus. If you develop COVID-19 symptoms, contact your healthcare provider, and tell them about your symptoms and your travel or exposure to a COVID-19 patient.
- For people who are ill with COVID-19, please follow CDC guidance on how to reduce the risk of spreading your illness to others (see pages 70–74).

How COVID-19 Spreads

Current understanding about how the virus that causes coronavirus disease 2019 (COVID-19) spreads is largely based on what is known about similar coronaviruses. COVID-19 is a new disease and there is more to learn about how it spreads, the severity of illness it causes, and to what extent it may spread in the United States.

Person-to-person spread

The virus is thought to spread mainly from person-to-person.
- Between people who are in close contact with one another (within about 6 feet).
- Through respiratory droplets produced when an infected person coughs or sneezes.

These droplets can land in the mouths or noses of people who are nearby or possibly be inhaled into the lungs.

Spread from contact with infected surfaces or objects

It may be possible that a person can get COVID-19 by touching a surface or object that has the virus on it and then touching their own mouth, nose, or possibly their eyes, but this is not thought to be the main way the virus spreads.

Can someone spread the virus without being sick?

- People are thought to be most contagious when they are most symptomatic (the sickest).
- Some spread might be possible before people show symptoms; there have been reports of this occurring with this new coronavirus, but this is not thought to be the main way the virus spreads.

How easily does the virus spread?

How easily a virus spreads from person-to-person can vary. Some viruses are highly contagious (spread easily), like measles, while other viruses do not spread as easily. Another factor is whether the spread is sustained.

The virus that causes COVID-19 seems to be spreading easily and sustainably in the community ("community spread") in some affected geographic areas. Community spread means people have been infected with the virus in an area, including some who are not sure how or where they became infected.

Symptoms

For confirmed coronavirus disease 2019 (COVID-19) cases, reported illnesses have ranged from mild symptoms to severe illness and death. Symptoms can include:

- Fever
- Cough
- Shortness of breath

CDC believes at this time that symptoms of COVID-19 may appear in as few as 2 days or as long as 14 days after exposure. This is based on what has been seen previously as the incubation period of MERS-CoV viruse.

Prevention & Treatment

Prevention

There is currently no vaccine to prevent coronavirus disease 2019 (COVID-19). The best way to prevent illness is to avoid being exposed to this virus. However, as a reminder, CDC always recommends everyday preventive actions to help prevent the spread of respiratory diseases, including:

- Avoid close contact with people who are sick.
- Avoid touching your eyes, nose, and mouth.
- Stay home when you are sick.
- Cover your cough or sneeze with a tissue, then throw the tissue in the trash.
- Clean and disinfect frequently touched objects and surfaces using a regular household cleaning spray or wipe.
- Follow CDC's recommendations for using a facemask.
  - CDC does not recommend that people who are well wear a facemask to protect themselves from respiratory diseases, including COVID-19.
  - Facemasks should be used by people who show symptoms of COVID-19 to help prevent the spread of the disease to others. The use of facemasks is also crucial for health workers and people who are taking care of someone in close settings (at home or in a health care facility).

Wash your hands often with soap and water for at least 20 seconds, especially after going to the bathroom; before eating; and after blowing your nose, coughing, or sneezing.

- If soap and water are not readily available, use an alcohol-based hand sanitizer with at least 60% alcohol. Always wash hands with soap and water if hands are visibly dirty.

These are everyday habits that can help prevent the spread of several viruses.

Treatment

There is no specific antiviral treatment recommended for COVID-19. People with COVID-19 should receive supportive care to help relieve symptoms. For severe cases, treatment should include care to support vital organ functions.

People who think they may have been exposed to COVID-19 should contact their healthcare provider immediately.

What to Do If You Are Sick With Coronavirus Disease 2019 (COVID-19)

If you develop a fever[1] and symptoms of respiratory illness, such as cough or shortness of breath, within 14 days after travel from China, you should call ahead to a healthcare professional and mention your recent travel or close contact. If you have had close contact[2] with someone showing these symptoms who has recent-

---

1   Fever may be subjective or confirmed
2   Close contact is defined as—
a) being within approximately 6 feet (2 meters) of a COVID-19 case for a prolonged period of time; close contact can occur while caring for, living with, visiting, or sharing a health care waiting area or room with a COVID-19 case

ly traveled from this area, you should call ahead to a healthcare professional and mention your close contact and their recent travel. Your healthcare professional will work with your state's public health department and CDC to determine if you need to be tested for COVID-19.

Steps to help prevent the spread of COVID-19 if you are sick

If you are sick with COVID-19 or suspect you are infected with the virus that causes COVID-19, follow the steps below to help prevent the disease from spreading to people in your home and community.

Stay home except to get medical care:

You should restrict activities outside your home, except for getting medical care. Do not go to work, school, or public areas. Avoid using public transportation, ride-sharing, or taxis.

Separate yourself from other people and animals in your home:

People: As much as possible, you should stay in a specific room and away from other people in your home. Also, you should use a separate bathroom, if available.

– or –

b) having direct contact with infectious secretions of a COVID-19 case (e.g., being coughed on). If such contact occurs while not wearing recommended personal protective equipment or PPE (e.g., gowns, gloves, NIOSH-certified disposable N95 respirator, eye protection), criteria for PUI consideration are met.

See CDC's updated Interim Healthcare Infection Prevention and Control Recommendations for Persons Under Investigation for 2019 Novel Coronavirus: https://www.cdc.gov/coronavirus/2019-ncov/infection-control/control-recommendations.html?CDC_AA_refVal=https%3A%2F%2Fwww.cdc.gov%2Fcoronavirus%2F2019-ncov%2Fhcp%2Finfection-control.html.

Data to inform the definition of close contact are limited. Considerations when assessing close contact include the duration of exposure (e.g., longer exposure time likely increases exposure risk) and the clinical symptoms of the person with COVID-19 (e.g., coughing likely increases exposure risk as does exposure to a severely ill patient). Special consideration should be given to those exposed in health care settings.

Animals: You should restrict contact with pets and other animals while you are sick with COVID-19, just like you would around other people. Although there have not been reports of pets or other animals becoming sick with COVID-19, it is still recommended that people sick with COVID-19 limit contact with animals until more information is known about the virus. When possible, have another member of your household care for your animals while you are sick. If you are sick with COVID-19, avoid contact with your pet, including petting, snuggling, being kissed or licked, and sharing food. If you must care for your pet or be around animals while you are sick, wash your hands before and after you interact with pets and wear a facemask.

Call ahead before visiting your doctor:

If you have a medical appointment, call the healthcare provider and tell them that you have or may have COVID-19. This will help the healthcare provider's office take steps to keep other people from getting infected or exposed.

Wear a facemask:

You should wear a facemask when you are around other people (e.g., sharing a room or vehicle) or pets and before you enter a healthcare provider's office. If you are not able to wear a facemask (for example, because it causes trouble breathing), then people who live with you should not stay in the same room with you, or they should wear a facemask if they enter your room.

Cover your coughs and sneezes:

Cover your mouth and nose with a tissue when you cough or sneeze. Throw used tissues in a lined trash can; immediately wash your hands with soap and water for at least 20 seconds or clean your hands with an alcohol-based hand sanitizer that contains 60 to 95% alcohol, covering all surfaces of your hands and rubbing them together until they feel dry. Soap and water should be used preferentially if hands are visibly dirty.

Clean your hands often:

Wash your hands often with soap and water for at least 20 seconds or clean your hands with an alcohol-based hand sanitizer that contains 60 to 95% alcohol, covering all surfaces of your hands and rubbing them together until they feel dry. Soap and water should be used preferentially if hands are visibly dirty. Avoid touching your eyes, nose, and mouth with unwashed hands.

Avoid sharing personal household items:

You should not share dishes, drinking glasses, cups, eating utensils, towels, or bedding with other people or pets in your home. After using these items, they should be washed thoroughly with soap and water.

Clean all "high-touch" surfaces everyday:

High touch surfaces include counters, tabletops, doorknobs, bathroom fixtures, toilets, phones, keyboards, tablets, and bedside tables. Also, clean any surfaces that may have blood, stool, or body fluids on them. Use a household cleaning spray or wipe, according to the label instructions. Labels contain instructions for safe and effective use of the cleaning product including precautions you should take when applying the product, such as wearing gloves and making sure you have good ventilation during use of the product.

Monitor your symptoms:

Seek prompt medical attention if your illness is worsening (e.g., difficulty breathing). **Before** seeking care, call your healthcare provider and tell them that you have, or are being evaluated for, COVID-19. Put on a facemask before you enter the facility. These steps will help the healthcare provider's office to keep other people in the office or waiting room from getting infected or exposed. Ask your healthcare provider to call the local or state health department. Persons who are placed under active monitoring or facilitated self-monitoring should follow instructions provided by their local health department or occupational health professionals, as appropriate.

If you have a medical emergency and need to call 911, notify the dispatch personnel that you have, or are being evaluated for COVID-19. If possible, put on a facemask before emergency medical services arrive.

Discontinuing home isolation

Patients with confirmed COVID-19 should remain under home isolation precautions until the risk of secondary transmission to others is thought to be low. The decision to discontinue home isolation precautions should be made on a case-by-case basis, in consultation with healthcare providers and state and local health departments.

Stigma Related to COVID-19

The risk of getting coronavirus disease 2019 is currently low in the U.S. due in part to quick action from health authorities. However, some people are worried about the disease. Fear and anxiety can lead to social stigma towards Chinese or other Asian Americans. Stigma and discrimination can occur when people associate an infectious disease, such as COVID-19, with a population or nationality, even though not everyone in that population or from that region is specifically at risk for the disease (for example, Chinese-Americans and other Asian-Americans living in the United States).

Stigma hurts everyone by creating more fear or anger towards ordinary people instead of the disease that is causing the problem. We can fight stigma and help not hurt others by providing social support. We can communicate the facts that being Chinese or Asian American does not increase the chance of getting or spreading COVID-19.

People—including those of Asian descent—who have not recently traveled to China or been in contact with a person who is a confirmed or suspected case of COVID-19 are not at greater risk of acquiring and spreading COVID-19 than other Americans.

- Viruses cannot target people from specific populations, ethnicities, or racial backgrounds.
- People from China in the U.S. may be worried or anxious about friends and relatives who are living in the region. Facing stigma can make fear and anxiety worsen. Social support during this outbreak can help them cope.

People who have returned from China more than 14 days ago and do not have symptoms are not infected with the virus and contact with them will not give you the virus.

- People who have traveled to areas where the COVID-19 outbreak is happening to help have performed a valuable service to everyone by helping make sure this disease does not spread further.
- Helping fight an outbreak can be mentally and emotionally challenging. These helpers need social support upon their return.
- The U.S. government has taken unprecedented steps related to travel in response to the growing public health threat posed by this new coronavirus, including suspending entry in the United States of foreign nationals who have visited China within the past 14 days. Measures to detect this virus among those who are allowed entry into the United States (U.S. citizens, residents and family) who have been in China within 14 days also are being implemented.

Communicators and public health officials can help counter stigma during the COVID-19 response.

- Maintain privacy and confidentiality of those seeking health care and those who may be part of any contact investigation.
- Timely communication of the risk or lack of risk from associations with products, people, and places.
- Raise awareness about COVID-19 without increasing fear.
- Share accurate information about how the virus spreads.
- Speak out against negative behaviors, including negative statements on social media about groups of people, or exclusion of people who pose no risk from regular activities.
- Be cautious about the images that are shared. Make sure they do not reinforce stereotypes.
- Engage with stigmatized groups in person and through media channels including news media and social media.
- Share the need for social support for people who have returned from China or are worried about friends or relatives in the affected region.

Share Facts About COVID-19

Know the facts about coronavirus disease 2019 (COVID-19) and help stop the spread of rumors.

For up-to-date information, visit CDC's coronavirus disease 2019 situation summary page https://www.cdc.gov/coronavirus/2019-ncov/summary.html.

Fact 1: Diseases can make anyone sick regardless of their race or ethnicity.

People of Asian descent, including Chinese Americans, are not more likely to get COVID-19 than any other American. Help stop fear by letting people know that being of Asian descent does not increase the chance of getting or spreading COVID-19.

Fact 2: The risk of getting COVID-19 in the U.S. is currently low.

Some people who have traveled to places where many people have gotten sick with COVID-19 may be monitored by health officials to protect their health and the health of other people in the community.

Fact 3: Someone who has completed quarantine or has been released from isolation does not pose a risk of infection to other people.

For up-to-date information, visit CDC's coronavirus disease situation summary page https://www.cdc.gov/coronavirus/2019-ncov/summary.html.

Fact 4: You can help stop COVID-19 by knowing the signs and symptoms:

- Fever
- Cough
- Shortness of breath

Seek medical advice if you have traveled to China in the past 14 days and feel sick. Call ahead before you go to a doctor's office or emergency room. Tell them about your recent travel and your symptoms.

Fact 5: There are simple things you can do to help keep yourself and others healthy.

- Wash your hands often with soap and water for at least 20 seconds, especially after going to the bathroom; before eating; and after blowing your nose, coughing, or sneezing.

- Avoid touching your eyes, nose, and mouth with unwashed hands.
- Stay home when you are sick.
- Cover your cough or sneeze with a tissue, then throw the tissue in the trash.

Disease Basics

Q: What is a novel coronavirus?

A: A novel coronavirus is a new coronavirus that has not been previously identified. The virus causing coronavirus disease 2019 (COVID-19), is not the same as the coronaviruses that commonly circulate among humans and cause mild illness, like the common cold.

A diagnosis with coronavirus 229E, NL63, OC43, or HKU1 is not the same as a COVID-19 diagnosis. Patients with COVID-19 will be evaluated and cared for differently than patients with common coronavirus diagnosis.

Q: Why is the disease causing the outbreak now being called coronavirus disease 2019, COVID-19?

A: On February 11, 2020 the World Health Organization announced an official name for the disease that is causing the 2019 novel coronavirus outbreak, first identified in Wuhan China. The new name of this disease is coronavirus disease 2019, abbreviated as COVID-19. In COVID-19, 'CO' stands for 'corona,' 'VI' for 'virus,' and 'D' for disease. Formerly, this disease was referred to as "2019 novel coronavirus" or "2019-nCoV."

There are many types of human coronaviruses including some that commonly cause mild upper-respiratory tract illnesses. COVID-19 is a new disease, caused be a novel (or new) coronavirus that has not previously been seen in humans. The name of this disease was selected following the World Health Organization (WHO) best practice for naming of new human nfectious diseases.

Q: What is the name of the virus causing the outbreak of coronavirus disease starting in 2019?

A: On February 11, 2020, the International Committee on Taxonomy of Viruses, charged with naming new viruses, named the novel coronavirus, first identified in Wuhan, China, severe acute respiratory syndrome coronavirus 2, shortened to SARS-CoV-2.

As the name indicates, the virus is related to the SARS-associated coronavirus (SARS-CoV) that caused an outbreak of severe acute respiratory syndrome (SARS) in 2002-2003, however it is not the same virus.

Q: What is the source of COVID-19?

A: Coronaviruses are a large family of viruses. Some cause illness in people, and others, such as canine and feline coronaviruses, only infect animals. Rarely, animal coronaviruses that infect animals have emerged to infect people and can spread between people. This is suspected to have occurred for the virus that causes COVID-19. Middle East Respiratory Syndrome (MERS) and Severe Acute Respiratory Syndrome (SARS) are two other examples of coronaviruses that originated from animals and then spread to people.

Q: How does the virus causing Coronavirus Disease-2019 (COVID-19), spread?

A: This virus was first detected in Wuhan City, Hubei Province, China. The first infections were linked to a live animal market, but the virus is now spreading from person-to-person. It's important to note that person-to-person spread can happen on a continuum. Some viruses are highly contagious (like measles), while other viruses are less so. Currently, it's unclear how easily or sustainably this virus is spreading between people.

Q: Can someone who has had COVID-19 spread the illness to others?

A: The virus that causes COVID-19 is spreading from person-to-person. Someone who is actively sick with COVID-19 can spread the illness to others. That is why CDC recommends that these patients be isolated either in the hospital or at home (depending on how sick they are) until they are better and no longer pose a risk of infecting others.

How long someone is actively sick can vary so the decision on when to release someone from isolation is made on a case-by-case basis in consultation with doctors, infection prevention and control experts, and public health officials and involves considering specifics of each situation including disease severity, illness signs and symptoms, and results of laboratory testing for that patient.

Current CDC guidance for when it is OK to release someone from isolation is made on a case by case basis and includes meeting all of the following requirements:

- The patient is free from fever without the use of fever-reducing medications.
- The patient is no longer showing symptoms, including cough.
- The patient has tested negative on at least two consecutive respiratory specimens collected at least 24 hours apart.

Someone who has been released from isolation is not considered to pose a risk of infection to others.

Q: Can someone who has been quarantined for COVID-19 spread the illness to others?

A: Quarantine means separating a person or group of people who have been exposed to a contagious disease but have not developed illness (symptoms) from others who have not been exposed, in order to prevent the possible spread of that disease. Quarantine is usually established for the incubation period of the communicable disease, which is the span of time during which people have developed illness after exposure. For COVID-19, the period of quarantine is 14 days from the last date of exposure, because 14 days is the longest incubation period seen for similar coronaviruses. Someone who has been released from COVID-19 quarantine is not considered a risk for spreading the virus to others because they have not developed illness during the incubation period.

Q: Why might someone blame or avoid individuals and groups (create stigma) because of COVID-19?

A. People in the U.S. may be worried or anxious about friends and relatives who are living in or visiting areas where COVID-19 is spreading. Some people are worried about the disease. Fear and anxiety can lead to social stigma, for example, towards Chinese or other Asian Americans or people who were in quarantine.

Stigma is discrimination against an identifiable group of people, a place, or a nation. Stigma is associated with a lack of knowledge about how COVID-19 spreads, a need to blame someone, fears about disease and death, and gossip that spreads rumors and myths.

Stigma hurts everyone by creating more fear or anger towards ordinary people instead of the disease that is causing the problem.

Q: How can people help stop stigma related to COVID-19?

A: People can fight stigma and help, not hurt, others by providing social support. Counter stigma by learning and sharing facts. Communicating the facts that viruses do not target specific racial or ethnic groups and how COVID-19 actually spreads can help stop stigma.

Q: Is the coronavirus that causes COVID-19 the same as the MERS-CoV or the SARS-CoV virus?

A: No. Coronaviruses are a large family of viruses. Some coronaviruses cause cold-like illnesses in people. Others cause illness in certain types of animals, such as cattle, camels and bats. Rarely, animal coronaviruses can spread to people. This happened with SARS-CoV and MERS-CoV. The virus that causes COVID-19 likely also originated in an animal and spread to humans. The coronavirus most similar to the virus causing COVID-19 is SARS-CoV. There are ongoing investigations to learn more. The situation is changing, and information will be updated as it becomes available.

Prevention

Q: How can I help protect myself?

A: See page 69 to learn about how to protect yourself from respiratory illnesses, like COVID-19.

Q: What should I do if I had close contact with someone who has COVID-19?

A: Household members, intimate partners, and caregivers in a non-healthcare setting may have close contact with a person with symptomatic, laboratory-confirmed COVID-19 or a person under investigation. Close contacts should monitor their health; they should call their healthcare provider right away if they develop symptoms suggestive of COVID-19 (e.g., fever, cough, shortness of breath).
Close contacts should also follow these recommendations:

- Make sure that you understand and can help the patient follow their healthcare provider's instructions for medication(s) and care. You should help the patient with basic needs in the home and provide support for getting groceries, prescriptions, and other personal needs.
- Monitor the patient's symptoms. If the patient is getting sicker, call his or her healthcare provider and tell them that the patient has laboratory-confirmed COVID-19. This will help the healthcare provider's office take steps to keep

other people in the office or waiting room from getting infected. Ask the healthcare provider to call the local or state health department for additional guidance. If the patient has a medical emergency and you need to call 911, notify the dispatch personnel that the patient has, or is being evaluated for COVID-19.

- Household members should stay in another room or be separated from the patient as much as possible. Household members should use a separate bedroom and bathroom, if available.
- Prohibit visitors who do not have an essential need to be in the home.
- Household members should care for any pets in the home. Do not handle pets or other animals while sick. For more information, see COVID-19 and Animals.
- Make sure that shared spaces in the home have good air flow, such as by an air conditioner or an opened window, weather permitting.
- Perform hand hygiene frequently. Wash your hands often with soap and water for at least 20 seconds or use an alcohol-based hand sanitizer that contains 60 to 95% alcohol, covering all surfaces of your hands and rubbing them together until they feel dry. Soap and water should be used preferentially if hands are visibly dirty.
- Avoid touching your eyes, nose, and mouth with unwashed hands.
- You and the patient should wear a facemask if you are in the same room.
- Wear a disposable facemask and gloves when you touch or have contact with the patient's blood, stool, or body fluids, such as saliva, sputum, nasal mucus, vomit, urine.
  - Throw out disposable facemasks and gloves after using them. Do not reuse.
  - When removing personal protective equipment, first remove and dispose of gloves. Then, immediately clean your hands with soap and water or alcohol-based hand sanitizer. Next, remove and dispose of facemask, and

immediately clean your hands again with soap and water or alcohol-based hand sanitizer.

- Avoid sharing household items with the patient. You should not share dishes, drinking glasses, cups, eating utensils, towels, bedding, or other items. After the patient uses these items, you should wash them thoroughly (see below "Wash laundry thoroughly").

- Clean all "high-touch" surfaces, such as counters, tabletops, doorknobs, bathroom fixtures, toilets, phones, keyboards, tablets, and bedside tables, every day. Also, clean any surfaces that may have blood, stool, or body fluids on them.

- Use a household cleaning spray or wipe, according to the label instructions. Labels contain instructions for safe and effective use of the cleaning product including precautions you should take when applying the product, such as wearing gloves and making sure you have good ventilation during use of the product.

- Wash laundry thoroughly.

- Immediately remove and wash clothes or bedding that have blood, stool, or body fluids on them.

- Wear disposable gloves while handling soiled items and keep soiled items away from your body. Clean your hands (with soap and water or an alcohol-based hand sanitizer) immediately after removing your gloves.

- Read and follow directions on labels of laundry or clothing items and detergent. In general, using a normal laundry detergent according to washing machine instructions and dry thoroughly using the warmest temperatures recommended on the clothing label.

- Place all used disposable gloves, facemasks, and other contaminated items in a lined container before disposing of them with other household waste. Clean your hands (with soap and water or an alcohol-based hand sanitizer) immediately after handling these items. Soap and water should be used preferentially if hands are visibly dirty.

- Discuss any additional questions with your state or local health department or healthcare provider.

Q: Does CDC recommend the use of facemask in the community to prevent COVID-19?

A: CDC does not recommend that people who are well wear a facemask to protect themselves from respiratory illnesses, including COVID-19. You should only wear a mask if a healthcare professional recommends it. A facemask should be used by people who have COVID-19 and are showing symptoms. This is to protect others from the risk of getting infected. The use of facemasks also is crucial for health workers and other people who are taking care of someone infected with COVID-19 in close settings (at home or in a health care facility).

Medical Information

Q: What are the symptoms and complications that COVID-19 can cause?

A: Current symptoms reported for patients with COVID-19 have included mild to severe respiratory illness with fever[3], cough, and difficulty breathing.

Q: Should I be tested for COVID-19?

A: If you develop a fever and symptoms of respiratory illness, such as cough or shortness of breath, within 14 days after travel from China, you should call ahead to a healthcare professional and mention your recent travel or close contact. If you have had close contact[4] with someone showing these symptoms who has recent-

---

3 Fever may be subjective or confirmed
4 Close contact is defined as—
a) being within approximately 6 feet (2 meters) of a COVID-19 case for a prolonged period of time; close contact can occur while caring for, living with, visiting, or sharing a health care waiting area or room with a COVID-19 case
– or –
b) having direct contact with infectious secretions of a COVID-19 case (e.g., being coughed on) *(note continued on next page)*

ly traveled from this area, you should call ahead to a healthcare professional and mention your close contact and their recent travel. Your healthcare professional will work with your state's public health department and CDC to determine if you need to be tested for COVID-19.

Q: How do you test a person for COVID-19?

A: At this time, diagnostic testing for COVID-19 can be conducted only at CDC.

State and local health departments who have identified a person under investigation (PUI) should immediately notify CDC's Emergency Operations Center (EOC) to report the PUI and determine whether testing for COVID-19 at CDC is indicated. The EOC will assist local/state health departments to collect, store, and ship specimens appropriately to CDC, including during afterhours or on weekends/holidays.

Q: Can a person test negative and later test positive for COVID-19?

A: Using the CDC-developed diagnostic test, a negative result means that the virus that causes COVID-19 was not found in the person's sample. In the early stages of infection, it is possible the virus will not be detected.

If such contact occurs while not wearing recommended personal protective equipment or PPE (e.g., gowns, gloves, NIOSH-certified disposable N95 respirator, eye protection), criteria for PUI consideration are met"

See CDC's updated Interim Healthcare Infection Prevention and Control Recommendations for Persons Under Investigation for 2019 Novel Coronavirus: https://www.cdc.gov/coronavirus/2019-ncov/infection-control/control-recommendations.html?CDC_AA_refVal=https%3A%2F%2Fwww.cdc.gov%2Fcoronavirus%2F2019-ncov%2Fhcp%2Finfection-control.html.

Data to inform the definition of close contact are limited. Considerations when assessing close contact include the duration of exposure (e.g., longer exposure time likely increases exposure risk) and the clinical symptoms of the person with COVID-19 (e.g., coughing likely increases exposure risk as does exposure to a severely ill patient). Special consideration should be given to those exposed in health care settings.

For COVID-19, a negative test result for a sample collected while a person has symptoms likely means that the COVID-19 virus is not causing their current illness.

Q: What should healthcare professionals and health departments do?

A: For recommendations and guidance on persons under investigation; infection control, including personal protective equipment guidance; home care and isolation; and case investigation, see Information for Healthcare Professionals: https://www.cdc.gov/coronavirus/2019-nCoV/hcp/clinical-criteria.html. For information on specimen collection and shipment, see Information for Laboratories: https://www.cdc.gov/coronavirus/2019-nCoV/lab/index.html For information for public health professional on COVID-19, see Information for Public Health Professionals: https://www.cdc.gov/coronavirus/2019-ncov/php/index.html.

Information on COVID-19 and Pregnant Women and Children

There is not currently information from published scientific reports about susceptibility of pregnant women to COVID-19. Pregnant women experience immunologic and physiologic changes which might make them more susceptible to viral respiratory infections, including COVID-19.

There is no evidence that children are more susceptible to COVID-19. In fact, most confirmed cases of COVID-19 reported from China have occurred in adults. Infections in children have been reported, including in very young children. There is an ongoing investigation to determine more about this outbreak. This is a rapidly evolving situation and information will be updated as it becomes available. Information about children and pregnant women and COVID-19 is available on this page.

Frequently Asked Questions and Answers: Coronavirus Disease 2019 (COVID-19) and Pregnancy

Q: Are pregnant women more susceptible to infection, or at increased risk for severe illness, morbidity, or mortality with COVID-19, compared with the general public?

A: We do not have information from published scientific reports about susceptibility of pregnant women to COVID-19. Pregnant women experience immunologic and physiologic changes which might make them more susceptible to viral respiratory infections, including COVID-19. Pregnant women also might be at risk for severe illness, morbidity, or mortality compared to the general population as observed in cases of other related coronavirus infections [including severe acute respiratory syndrome coronavirus (SARS-CoV) and Middle East respiratory syndrome coronavirus (MERS-CoV)] and other viral respiratory infections, such as influenza, during pregnancy.

Though person-to-person spread of the virus that causes COVID-19 has been observed in the United States among close contacts, this virus is not currently spreading among persons in the community in the United States and the immediate risk to the general public is low. Pregnant women should engage in usual preventive actions to avoid infection like washing hands often and avoiding people who are sick.

Q: Are pregnant women with COVID-19 at increased risk for adverse pregnancy outcomes?

A: We do not have information on adverse pregnancy outcomes in pregnant women with COVID-19. Pregnancy loss, including miscarriage and stillbirth, has been observed in cases of infection with other related coronaviruses [SARS-CoV and MERS-CoV] during pregnancy. High fevers during the first trimester of pregnancy can increase the risk of certain birth defects.

Q: Are pregnant healthcare personnel at increased risk for adverse outcomes if they care for patients with COVID-19?

A: Pregnant healthcare personnel (HCP) should follow risk assessment and infection control guidelines for HCP exposed to patients with suspected or confirmed COVID-19. Adherence to recommended infection prevention and control practices is an important part of protecting all HCP in healthcare settings. Information on COVID-19 in pregnancy is very limited; facilities may want to consider limiting exposure of pregnant HCP to patients with confirmed or suspected COVID-19, especially during higher risk procedures (e.g., aerosol-generating procedures) if feasible based on staffing availability.

Q: Can pregnant women with COVID-19 pass the virus to their fetus or newborn (i.e. vertical transmission)?

A: The virus that causes COVID-19 is thought to spread mainly by close contact with an infected person through respiratory droplets. Whether a pregnant woman with COVID-19 can transmit the virus that causes COVID-19 to her fetus or neonate by other routes of vertical transmission (before, during, or after delivery) is still unknown. However, in limited recent case series of infants born to mothers with COVID-19 published in the peer-reviewed literature, none of the infants have tested positive for the virus that causes COVID-19. Additionally, virus was not detected in samples of amniotic fluid or breastmilk.

Limited information is available about vertical transmission for other coronaviruses (MERS-CoV and SARS-CoV) but vertical transmission has not been reported for these infections.

Q: Are infants born to mothers with COVID-19 during pregnancy at increased risk for adverse outcomes?

A: Based on limited case reports, adverse infant outcomes (e.g., preterm birth) have been reported among infants born to mothers positive for COVID-19 during pregnancy. However, it is not clear that these outcomes were related to maternal infection, and at this time the risk of adverse infant outcomes is not known. Given the limited data available related to COVID-19 during pregnancy, knowledge of adverse outcomes from other respiratory viral infections may provide some information. For example, other respiratory viral infections during pregnancy, such as influenza, have been associated with adverse neonatal outcomes, including low birth weight and preterm birth. Additionally, having a cold or influenza with high fever early in pregnancy may increase the risk of certain birth defects. Infants have been born preterm and/or small for gestational age to mothers with other coronavirus infections, SARS-CoV and MERS-CoV, during pregnancy.

Q: Is there a risk that COVID-19 in a pregnant woman or neonate could have long-term effects on infant health and development that may require clinical support beyond infancy?

A: At this time, there is no information on long-term health effects on infants either with COVID-19, or those exposed to the virus that causes COVID-19 in utero. In general, prematurity and low birth weight are associated with adverse long-term health effects.

Q: Is maternal illness with COVID-19 during lactation associated with potential risk to a breastfeeding infant?

A: Human-to-human transmission by close contact with a person with confirmed COVID-19 has been reported and is thought to occur mainly via respiratory droplets produced when a person with infection coughs or sneezes.

In limited case series reported to date, no evidence of virus has been found in the breast milk of women with COVID-19. No information is available on the transmission of the virus that causes COVID-19 through breast milk (i.e., whether infectious virus is present in the breast milk of an infected woman).

In limited reports of lactating women infected with SARS-CoV, virus has not been detected in breast milk; however, antibodies against SARS-CoV were detected in at least one sample.

Interim Guidance on Breastfeeding for a Mother Confirmed or Under Investigation for COVID-19

This interim guidance is intended for women who are confirmed to have COVID-19 or are persons-under-investigation (PUI) for COVID-19 and are currently breastfeeding. This interim guidance is based on what is currently known about COVID-19 and the transmission of other viral respiratory infections. CDC will update this interim guidance as needed as additional information becomes available. For breastfeeding guidance in the immediate postpartum setting, refer to https://www.cdc.gov/coronavirus/2019-ncov/hcp/inpatient-obstetric-healthcare-guidance.html.

Transmission of COVID-19 through breast milk

Much is unknown about how COVID-19 is spread. Person-to-person spread is thought to occur mainly via respiratory droplets produced when an infected person coughs or sneezes, similar to how influenza (flu) and other respiratory pathogens spread. In limited studies on women with COVID-19 and another coronavirus infection, Severe Acute Respiratory Syndrome (SARS-CoV), the virus has not been detected in breast milk; however we do not know whether mothers with COVID-19 can transmit the virus via breast milk.

CDC breastfeeding guidance for other infectious illnesses

Breast milk provides protection against many illnesses. There are rare exceptions when breastfeeding or feeding expressed breast milk is not recommended. CDC has no specific guidance for breastfeeding during infection with similar viruses like SARS-CoV or Middle Eastern Respiratory Syndrome (MERS-CoV).

Outside of the immediate postpartum setting, CDC recommends that a mother with flu continue breastfeeding or feeding expressed breast milk to her infant while taking precautions to avoid spreading the virus to her infant.

Guidance on breastfeeding for mothers with confirmed COVID-19 or under investigation for COVID-19

Breast milk is the best source of nutrition for most infants. However, much is unknown about COVID-19. Whether and how to start or continue breastfeeding should be determined by the mother in coordination with her family and healthcare providers. A mother with confirmed COVID-19 or who is a symptomatic PUI should take all possible precautions to avoid spreading the virus to her infant, including washing her hands before touching the infant and wearing a face mask, if possible, while feeding at the breast. If expressing breast milk with a manual or electric breast pump, the mother should wash her hands before touching any pump or bottle parts and follow recommendations for proper pump cleaning after each use. If possible, consider having someone who is well feed the expressed breast milk to the infant.

Frequently Asked Questions and Answers: Coronavirus Disease-2019 (COVID-19) and Children

Q: Are children more susceptible to the virus that causes COVID-19 compared with the general population and how can infection be prevented?

A: No, there is no evidence that children are more susceptible. In fact, most confirmed cases of COVID-19 reported from China have occurred in adults. Infections in children have been reported, including in very young children. From limited information published from past Severe Acute Respiratory Syndrome coronavirus (SARS-CoV) and Middle East respiratory syndrome coronavirus (MERS-CoV) outbreaks, infection among children was relatively uncommon.

Person-to-person spread of the virus that causes COVID-19 has been seen among close contacts of returned travelers from Hubei province in China. This virus is not currently spreading in the community in the United States and risk to the general public is low. Children should engage in usual preventive actions to avoid infection, including cleaning hands often using soap and water or alcohol-based hand sanitizer, avoiding people who are sick, and staying up to date on vaccinations, including influenza vaccine.

Q: Does the clinical presentation of COVID-19 differ in children compared with adults?

A: Limited reports of children with COVID-19 in China have described cold-like symptoms, such as fever, runny nose, and cough. Gastrointestinal symptoms (vomiting and diarrhea) have been reported in at least one child with COVID-19. These limited reports suggest that children with confirmed COVID-19 have generally presented with mild symptoms, and though severe complications (e.g., acute respiratory distress syndrome, septic shock) have been reported, they appear to be uncommon.

Q: Are children at increased risk for severe illness, morbidity, or mortality from COVID-19 infection compared with adults?

A: There have been very few reports of the clinical outcomes for children with COVID-19 to date. Limited reports from China suggest that children with confirmed COVID-19 may present with mild symptoms and though severe complications (e.g., acute respiratory distress syndrome, septic shock) have been reported, they appear to be uncommon. However, as with other respiratory illnesses, certain populations of children may be at increased risk of severe infection, such as children with underlying health conditions.

Q: Are there any treatments available for children with COVID-19?

A: There are currently no antiviral drugs recommended or licensed by the U.S. Food and Drug Administration for COVID-19. Clinical management includes prompt implementation of recommended infection prevention and control measures in healthcare settings and supportive management of complications.

Children and their family members should engage in usual preventive actions to prevent the spread of respiratory infections, including covering coughs, cleaning hands often with soap and water or alcohol-based hand sanitizer, and staying up to date on vaccinations, including influenza.

Interim Guidance for Businesses and Employers to Plan and Respond to Coronavirus Disease 2019 (COVID-19), February 2020

This interim guidance is based on what is currently known about the coronavirus disease 2019 (COVID-19). The Centers for Disease Control and Prevention (CDC) will update this interim guidance as needed and as additional information becomes available.

CDC is working across the Department of Health and Human Services and across the U.S. government in the public health response to COVID-19. Much is unknown about how the virus that causes COVID-19 spreads. Current knowledge is largely based on what is known about similar coronaviruses.

CDC Industry Guidance

- Resources for Airlines: https://www.cdc.gov/quarantine/air/managing-sick-travelers/ncov-airlines.html
- Resources for the Ship Industry: https://www.cdc.gov/quarantine/maritime/index.html

CDC Business Sector

Dr. Messonnier provides a situational update on COVID-19 for CDC private sector partners.

Coronaviruses are a large family of viruses that are common in humans and many different species of animals, including camels, cattle, cats, and bats. Rarely, animal coronaviruses can infect people and then spread between people, such as with MERS-CoV and SARS-CoV. The virus that causes COVID-19 is spreading from person-to-person in China and some limited person-to-person transmission has been reported in countries outside China, including the United States. However, respiratory illnesses like seasonal influenza, are currently widespread in many US communities.

The following interim guidance may help prevent workplace exposures to acute respiratory illnesses, including COVID-19, in non-healthcare settings. The guidance also provides planning considerations if there are more widespread, community outbreaks of COVID-19.

To prevent stigma and discrimination in the workplace, use only the guidance described below to determine risk of COVID-19. Do not make determinations of risk based on race or country of origin, and be sure to maintain confidentiality of people with confirmed COVID-29. There is much more to learn about the transmissibility, severity, and other features of COVID-19 and investigations are ongoing.

Recommended strategies for employers to use now:

- Actively encourage sick employees to stay home:
  - Employees who have symptoms of acute respiratory illness are recommended to stay home and not come to work until they are free of fever (100.4°F [37.8°C] or greater using an oral thermometer), signs of a fever, and any other symptoms for at least 24 hours, without the use of fever-reducing or other symptom-altering medicines (e.g. cough suppressants). Employees should notify their supervisor and stay home if they are sick.
  - Ensure that your sick leave policies are flexible and consistent with public health guidance and that employees are aware of these policies.
  - Talk with companies that provide your business with contract or temporary employees about the importance of sick employees staying home and encourage them to develop non-punitive leave policies.
  - Do not require a healthcare provider's note for employees who are sick with acute respiratory illness to validate their illness or to return to work, as healthcare provider offices and medical facilities may be extremely busy and not able to provide such documentation in a timely way.
  - Employers should maintain flexible policies that permit employees to stay home to care for a sick family member. Employers should be aware that more employees may need to stay at home to care for sick children or other sick family members than is usual.

- Separate sick employees:
  - CDC recommends that employees who appear to have acute respiratory illness symptoms (i.e. cough, shortness of breath) upon arrival to work or become sick during the day should be separated from other employees and be sent home immediately. Sick employees should cover their noses and mouths with a tissue when coughing or

sneezing (or an elbow or shoulder if no tissue is available).

- Emphasize staying home when sick, respiratory etiquette and hand hygiene by all employees:
  - Place posters that encourage staying home when sick, cough and sneeze etiquette, and hand hygiene at the entrance to your workplace and in other workplace areas where they are likely to be seen.
  - Provide tissues and no-touch disposal receptacles for use by employees.
  - Instruct employees to clean their hands often with an alcohol-based hand sanitizer that contains at least 60-95% alcohol, or wash their hands with soap and water for at least 20 seconds. Soap and water should be used preferentially if hands are visibly dirty.
  - Provide soap and water and alcohol-based hand rubs in the workplace. Ensure that adequate supplies are maintained. Place hand rubs in multiple locations or in conference rooms to encourage hand hygiene.
  - Visit the coughing and sneezing etiquette and clean hands webpage for more information: https://www.cdc.gov/healthywater/hygiene/etiquette/coughing_sneezing.html and https://www.cdc.gov/handwashing/materials.html.
- Perform routine environmental cleaning:
  - Routinely clean all frequently touched surfaces in the workplace, such as workstations, countertops, and doorknobs. Use the cleaning agents that are usually used in these areas and follow the directions on the label.
  - No additional disinfection beyond routine cleaning is recommended at this time.
  - Provide disposable wipes so that commonly used surfaces (for example, doorknobs, keyboards, remote controls, desks) can be wiped down by employees before each use.

- Advise employees before traveling to take certain steps:
  - Check the CDC's Traveler's Health Notices (https://wwwnc.cdc.gov/travel) for the latest guidance and recommendations for each country to which you will travel. Specific travel information for travelers going to and returning from China, and information for aircrew, can be found at on the CDC website: https://www.cdc.gov/coronavirus/2019-ncov/travelers/index.html.
  - Advise employees to check themselves for symptoms of acute respiratory illness (https://www.cdc.gov/coronavirus/-2019ncov/about/symptoms.html) before starting travel and notify their supervisor and stay home if they are sick.
  - Ensure employees who become sick while traveling or on temporary assignment understand that they should notify their supervisor and should promptly call a healthcare provider for advice if needed.
  - If outside the United States, sick employees should follow your company's policy for obtaining medical care or contact a healthcare provider or overseas medical assistance company to assist them with finding an appropriate healthcare provider in that country. A U.S. consular officer can help locate healthcare services. However, U.S. embassies, consulates, and military facilities do not have the legal authority, capability, and resources to evacuate or give medicines, vaccines, or medical care to private U.S. citizens overseas.
- Additional Measures in Response to Currently Occurring Sporadic Importations of the COVID-19:
  - Employees who are well but who have a sick family member at home with COVID-19 should notify their supervisor and refer to CDC guidance for how to conduct a risk assessment (https://www.cdc.gov/coronavirus/2019-ncov/php/risk-assessment.html) of their potential exposure.
  - If an employee is confirmed to have COVID-19, employers should inform fellow employees of their possible

exposure to COVID-19 in the workplace but maintain confidentiality as required by the Americans with Disabilities Act (ADA). Employees exposed to a co-worker with confirmed COVID-19 should refer to CDC guidance for how to conduct a risk assessment of their potential exposure.

Planning for a Possible COVID-19 Outbreak in the US

The severity of illness or how many people will fall ill from COVID-19 is unknown at this time. If there is evidence of a COVID-19 outbreak in the U.S., employers should plan to be able to respond in a flexible way to varying levels of severity and be prepared to refine their business response plans as needed. For the general American public, such as workers in non-healthcare settings and where it is unlikely that work tasks create an increased risk of exposures to COVID-19, the immediate health risk from COVID-19 is considered low. The CDC and its partners will continue to monitor national and international data on the severity of illness caused by COVID-19, will disseminate the results of these ongoing surveillance assessments, and will make additional recommendations as needed.

Planning Considerations

All employers need to consider how best to decrease the spread of acute respiratory illness and lower the impact of COVID-19 in their workplace in the event of an outbreak in the US. They should identify and communicate their objectives, which may include one or more of the following: (a) reducing transmission among staff, (b) protecting people who are at higher risk for adverse health complications, (c) maintaining business operations, and (d) minimizing adverse effects on other entities in their supply chains. Some of the key considerations when making decisions on appropriate responses are:

- Disease severity (i.e., number of people who are sick, hospitalization and death rates) in the community where the business is located;
- Impact of disease on employees that are vulnerable and may be at higher risk for COVID-19 adverse health complications. Inform employees that some people may be at higher risk for severe illness, such as older adults and those with chronic medical conditions.
- Prepare for possible increased numbers of employee absences due to illness in employees and their family members, dismissals of early childhood programs and K-12 schools due to high levels of absenteeism or illness:
  - Employers should plan to monitor and respond to absenteeism at the workplace. Implement plans to continue your essential business functions in case you experience higher than usual absenteeism.
  - Cross-train personnel to perform essential functions so that the workplace is able to operate even if key staff members are absent.
  - Assess your essential functions and the reliance that others and the community have on your services or products. Be prepared to change your business practices if needed to maintain critical operations (e.g., identify alternative suppliers, prioritize customers, or temporarily suspend some of your operations if needed).
- Employers with more than one business location are encouraged to provide local managers with the authority to take appropriate actions outlined in their business infectious disease outbreak response plan based on the condition in each locality.
- Coordination with state and local health officials is strongly encouraged for all businesses so that timely and accurate information can guide appropriate responses in each location where their operations reside. Since the intensity of an outbreak may differ according to geographic location, local health officials will be issuing guidance specific to their communities.

Important Considerations for Creating an Infectious Disease Outbreak Response Plan

All employers should be ready to implement strategies to protect their workforce from COVID-19 while ensuring continuity of operations. During a COVID-19 outbreak, all sick employees should stay home and away from the workplace, respiratory etiquette and hand hygiene should be encouraged, and routine cleaning of commonly touched surfaces should be performed regularly.

Employers should:

- Ensure the plan is flexible and involve your employees in developing and reviewing your plan.
- Conduct a focused discussion or exercise using your plan, to find out ahead of time whether the plan has gaps or problems that need to be corrected.
- Share your plan with employees and explain what human resources policies, workplace and leave flexibilities, and pay and benefits will be available to them.
- Share best practices with other businesses in your communities (especially those in your supply chain), chambers of commerce, and associations to improve community response efforts.

Recommendations for an Infectious Disease Outbreak Response Plan:

- Identify possible work-related exposure and health risks to your employees. OSHA has more information on how to protect workers from potential exposures: https://www.osha.gov/SLTC/covid19-/ to COVID-19.
- Review human resources policies to make sure that policies and practices are consistent with public health recommendations and are consistent with existing state and federal workplace laws (for more information on employer responsibilities, visit the Department of Labor's https://www.dol.gov/ and the Equal Employment Opportunity Commission's https://www.eeoc.gov/ websites).

- Explore whether you can establish policies and practices, such as flexible worksites (e.g., telecommuting) and flexible work hours (e.g., staggered shifts), to increase the physical distance among employees and between employees and others if state and local health authorities recommend the use of social distancing strategies. For employees who are able to telework, supervisors should encourage employees to telework instead of coming into the workplace until symptoms are completely resolved. Ensure that you have the information technology and infrastructure needed to support multiple employees who may be able to work from home.

- Identify essential business functions, essential jobs or roles, and critical elements within your supply chains (e.g., raw materials, suppliers, subcontractor services/products, and logistics) required to maintain business operations. Plan for how your business will operate if there is increasing absenteeism or these supply chains are interrupted.

- Set up authorities, triggers, and procedures for activating and terminating the company's infectious disease outbreak response plan, altering business operations (e.g., possibly changing or closing operations in affected areas), and transferring business knowledge to key employees. Work closely with your local health officials to identify these triggers.

- Plan to minimize exposure between employees and also between employees and the public, if public health officials call for social distancing.

- Establish a process to communicate information to employees and business partners on your infectious disease outbreak response plans and latest COVID-19 information. Anticipate employee fear, anxiety, rumors, and misinformation, and plan communications accordingly.

- In some communities, early childhood programs and K-12 schools may be dismissed, particularly if COVID-19 worsens. Determine how you will operate if absenteeism spikes from increases in sick employees, those who stay home to care for sick family members, and those who must stay home to watch their children if dismissed from school. Businesses and other employers should prepare to institute flexible workplace and leave policies for these employees.

- Local conditions will influence the decisions that public health officials make regarding community-level strategies; employers should take the time now to learn about plans in place in each community where they have a business.
- If there is evidence of a COVID-19 outbreak in the US, consider canceling non-essential business travel to additional countries per travel guidance on the CDC website (https://www.cdc.gov/coronavirus/-2019ncov/travelers/index.html).
  - Travel restrictions may be enacted by other countries which may limit the ability of employees to return home if they become sick while on travel status.
  - Consider cancelling large work-related meetings or events.
- Engage state and local health departments to confirm channels of communication and methods for dissemination of local outbreak information.

Community Mitigation Guidance for COVID-19 Response in the United States: Nonpharmaceutical Interventions for Community Preparedness and Outbreak Response

Nonpharmaceutical interventions (NPIs) are public health actions that can slow the spread of emerging respiratory diseases like COVID-19 for which vaccines and drug treatments are not yet available.[5] They include personal protective measures implemented by individuals and community measures implemented by affected communities. NPIs are used to build community preparedness in communities without known COVID-19 disease and to support outbreak responses in communities where local cases or cluster of diseases have occurred.

NPIS for Community Preparedness

CDC recommends individuals and families follow everyday preventive measures:

- Voluntary Home Isolation: Stay home when you are sick with respiratory disease symptoms. At the present time, these symptoms are more likely due to influenza or other respiratory viruses than to COVID-19-related virus.
- Respiratory Etiquette: Cover coughs and sneezes with a tissue, then throw it in the trash can.
- Hand Hygiene: Wash hands often with soap and water for at least 20 seconds; especially after going to the bathroom; before eating; and after blowing your nose, coughing, or sneezing.
- If soap and water are not readily available, use an alcohol-based hand sanitizer with 60%-95% alcohol.
- Environmental Health Action: Routinely clean frequently touched surfaces and objects

Routine use of these measures by individuals and their families will increase community resilience and readiness for responding to an outbreak.

---

5   Additional information about the evidence base for each NPI and considerations for their implementation is available in: Community Mitigation Guidelines to Prevent Pandemic Influenza — United States, 2017 https://www.cdc.gov/mmwr/volumes/66/rr/rr6601a1.htm#T1_down

NPIs for COVID-19 Outbreaks in Communities

- **Personal Protective Measures.** During an outbreak in your community, CDC recommends the everyday preventive measures listed above—especially *staying home when sick*—and taking these additional measures:
  - Keeping away from others who are sick.
  - Limiting face-to-face contact with others as much as possible
  - Consulting with your healthcare provider if you or your household members are at high risk for COVID-19 complications
  - Wearing a facemask if advised to do so by your healthcare provider or by a public health official
  - Staying home when a household member is sick with respiratory disease symptoms, if instructed to do so by public health officials or a health care provider (Voluntary Home Quarantine)
- **Community Measures.** If COVID-19 disease is occurring in your community, state and local public health authorities may decide to implement:
  - Temporary closures or dismissals of childcare facilities and schools
  - Other social distancing measures that increase the physical space between people, including:
    - Workplace social distancing measures, such as replacing in-person meetings with teleworking
    - Modifying, postponing, or cancelling mass gatherings.

Decisions about the implementation of community measures will be made by local and state officials, in consultation with federal officials as appropriate, and based on the scope of the outbreak and the severity of illness. Implementation will require extensive community engagement and ongoing and transparent public health communications.

COVID-19 and Animals

Q: What risks do animals or animal products imported from China pose?

A: CDC does not have any evidence to suggest that animals or animal products imported from China pose a risk for spreading COVID-19 in the United States. This is a rapidly evolving situation and information will be updated as it becomes available. The U.S. Centers for Disease Control and Prevention (CDC), the U.S. Department of Agriculture (USDA), and the U.S. Fish and Wildlife Service (FWS) play distinct but complementary roles in regulating the importation of live animals and animal products into the United States. CDC regulates animals and animal products that pose a threat to human health, USDA regulates animals and animal products that pose a threat to agriculture; and FWS regulates importation of endangered species and wildlife that can harm the health and welfare of humans, the interests of agriculture, horticulture, or forestry, and the welfare and survival of wildlife resources.

Q: Can I travel to the United States with pets during the COVID-19 outbreak?

A: Please refer to CDC's requirements for bringing a dog to the United States (https://www.cdc.gov/importation/bringing-an-animal-into-the-united-states/index.html). The current requirements for rabies vaccination apply to dogs imported from China, a high-risk country for rabies.

Q: Should I be concerned about pets or other animals and COVID-19?

A: While this virus seems to have emerged from an animal source, it is now spreading from person-to-person in China. There is no reason to think that any animals including pets in the United States might be a source of infection with this new coronavirus. To date,

CDC has not received any reports of pets or other animals becoming sick with COVID-19. At this time, there is no evidence that companion animals including pets can be infected with or spread COVID-19. However, since animals can spread other diseases to people, it's always a good idea to wash your hands after being around animals. For more information on the many benefits of pet ownership, as well as staying safe and healthy around animals including pets, livestock, and wildlife, visit CDC's Healthy Pets, Healthy People website (https://www.cdc.gov/healthypets/index.html).

Q: Should I avoid contact with pets or other animals if I am sick with COVID-19?

A: You should restrict contact with pets and other animals while you are sick with COVID-19, just like you would around other people. Although there have not been reports of pets or other animals becoming sick with COVID-19, it is still recommended that people sick with COVID-19 limit contact with animals until more information is known about the virus. When possible, have another member of your household care for your animals while you are sick. If you are sick with COVID-19, avoid contact with your pet, including petting, snuggling, being kissed or licked, and sharing food. If you must care for your pet or be around animals while you are sick, wash your hands before and after you interact with pets and wear a facemask.

Q: What precautions should be taken for animals that have recently been imported (for example, by shelters, rescue groups, or as personal pets) from China?

A: Animals imported from China will need to meet CDC and USDA requirements for entering the United States. At this time, there is no evidence that companion animals including pets can be infected with or spread COVID-19. As with any animal introduced to a new environment, animals recently imported from China should be observed daily for signs of illness. If an animal becomes ill, the animal should be examined by a veterinarian. Call your local veterinary clinic before bringing the animal into the clinic and let them know that the animal was recently in China.

Q: Should I avoid animals and animal markets while I am travelling?

A: In the United States, there is no reason to think that any animals, including pets or livestock, might be a source of COVID-19 infection at this time. If you are visiting a live animal market anywhere in the world, it is important to clean your hands thoroughly with soap and water before and after visiting the market. Avoid contact with sick animals or spoiled products, as well as contaminated fluids and waste.

Resources

CDC Coronavirus Disease 2019 (COVID-19) Situation Summary: https://www.cdc.gov/coronavirus/2019-ncov/summary.html

Interim Guidance for Administrators of US Childcare Programs and K-12 Schools to Plan, Prepare, and Respond to Coronavirus Disease 2019 (COVID-19): https://www.cdc.gov/mmwr/volumes/66/rr/rr6601a1.htm#T1_down

Interim Guidance for Businesses and Employers to Plan and Respond to Coronavirus Disease 2019 (COVID-19): https://www.cdc.gov/coronavirus/2019-ncov/specific-groups/guidance-business-response.html

CDC in Action: Preparing Communities for Potential Spread of COVID-19 https://www.cdc.gov/coronavirus/2019-ncov/php/preparing-communities.html

Notes

Use the following pages to record important information, list essential phone numbers, or to track symptoms or wellness protocols.